AIR FRYER

Bake Quickly With Your Air Fryer and Lose Weight!

(Best Recipes for Beginners and Food Lovers)

Eric Korn

Published by Alex Howard

© **Eric Korn**

All Rights Reserved

Air Fryer: Bake Quickly With Your Air Fryer and Lose Weight! (Best Recipes for Beginners and Food Lovers)

ISBN 978-1-989891-83-4

All rights reserved. No part of this guide may be reproduced in any form without permission in writing from the publisher except in the case of brief quotations embodied in critical articles or reviews.

Legal & Disclaimer

The information contained in this book is not designed to replace or take the place of any form of medicine or professional medical advice. The information in this book has been provided for educational and entertainment purposes only.

The information contained in this book has been compiled from sources deemed reliable, and it is accurate to the best of the Author's knowledge; however, the Author cannot guarantee its accuracy and validity and cannot be held liable for any errors or omissions. Changes are periodically made to this book. You must consult your doctor or get professional medical advice before using any of the suggested remedies, techniques, or information in this book.

Table of Contents

Part 1 1
Appetizers 2
Recipe #1 – Air Fried Onion Rings 2
Recipe #2 – Air-Fried Heart of Palms 3
Recipe #3 – Air Fried Spinach Leaves 4
Recipe #4 - Cheese Sticks 4
Recipe #5 – All Vegetable Fritters 6
Breakfast Recipes 7
Recipe #6 - Cheesy Ham and Egg in Potato Crust 7
Recipe #7 – Air Fryer Hash Browns 8
Recipe #8 - Air-Fried Spinach Eggs 10
Recipe #9 – Onion and Mushrooms Frittata 11
Recipe #10 – Cheesy Sunny Side Up 12
Recipe #11 – Carrots and Potatoes Frittata 13
Recipe #12 - Tuna Cheese Sandwich 14
Recipe #13 - Potatoes Gratin 15
Recipe #14 - Scrambled Eggs On Toast 16
Recipe #15 – Cheesy Zucchini Omelet 18
Recipe #16 - Tomato Leeks Frittata 19
Recipe #17 – Golden Bacon Cheese Rolls 20
Recipe #18 - Feta Cheese Triangles 21

Recipe #19 - Fried Plantains with Coconut Almond Flakes 22

Recipe #20 - Potato Wedges 23

Lunch Recipes 25

Recipe #21 Tuna Steaks with Spicy Cauliflower Pops 25

Recipe #22 - Shirataki Curry Noodle 27

Recipe #23 – Tomato Meatballs with Roasted Onions and Peppers 29

Recipe #24 - Beef Tenderloin with Sautéed Onions and Peppers 31

Recipe #25 – Air Fried Beef Meatballs in Tomato Sauce 32

Recipe #26 – Country-Style Chicken 33

Recipe #27 – Air Fried Asian Bok Choy 34

Recipe #28 - Cajun-Style Shrimp 35

Recipe #29 - Chili Crab Legs 37

Recipe #30 – Air Fried Baby Back Ribs 38

Recipe #31 – Citrusy Buttered Tilapia 39

Recipe #32 - Chicken Fries with Grilled Tomatoes 40

Recipe #33 - Chicken Skewer 42

Recipe #34 – Air Fried Pork Tenderloin 43

Bonus Lunch Recipes 44

Moroccan Meatballs with Mint Yogurt 44

Crusted Lamb 46

Creamy Chicken Mushrooms 47

Mushroom Chickpea Burger 48

Dinner Recipes 51

Recipe #35 – Air Fried Homemade Chicken Nuggets 51

Recipe #36 - Steak with Sausage Gravy and Potatoes 52

Recipe #37 - Beef Curry on Bed of Rice and Veggies 53

Recipe #38 – Fried Salmon Fillets with Kale Chips 55

Recipe #39 – Pepperoni Pizza Rolls 57

Recipe #40 – Air Fried Pork and Potatoes 58

Recipe #41 – Air Fried Beef Dumplings 59

Recipe #42 - Chicken with Cauliflower 61

Recipe #43 – Air Fried Coconut Shrimp 63

Recipe #44 - Turkey with Basil Pesto Tomatoes 64

Recipe #45 – Air Fried Aubergines and Tomatoes 65

Recipe #46 - Stuffed Garlic Mushrooms 67

Bonus Recipes 68

Shrimps with Vegetables Roast 68

Bonus Recipe - Almond-Crusted Chicken Slivers 70

Teriyaki Fish Steak 72

Snacks and Desserts 73

Recipe #47 – Zucchini Rolls 73

Recipe #48 - Doughnuts with Glaze 74

Recipe #49 – Air Fried Chocolate Cake with Apricot Jam 75

Recipe #50 - Apricot and Blueberries Crumble 77

Recipe #51 - Mushroom Chicken Spring Rolls 78

Recipe #52 – Raspberry Choco Cake 79

Recipe #53 - Pepperoni Patties 80

Recipe #54 - Raspberry Cheesecake Rolls 81

Recipe #55 – Air Fried Cheesy and Meaty Potato Skins 82

Recipe #56 – Air Fried Pork Cracklings 84

Recipe #57 - Soufflé 85

Recipe #58 - Pumpkin and Maple Cupcakes 86

Recipe #59 - Corn Rolls 88

Recipe #60 - Falafel with Cashew 90

Bonus Recipe 91

Pork and Shrimp Siomai 91

Sweet and Spicy Potato Sticks 93

Conclusion	95
Part 2	96
Introduction	97
Cooking Measurement Conversion Chart	99
Breakfast Recipes	100
Baked Eggs in Avocado Nests	100
Fried Eggs with Ham	101
Air Fryer Spinach Frittata	103
Easy Breakfast Casserole	105
French Toast Sticks	106
Side & Entrees	108
Green Beans with Shallots and Almonds	108
Fried Carrots with Cumin	109
Cheesy French Fries	110
Spinach with Bacon, Onion & Garlic	111
Feta Pillows	112
Asparagus Spears Rolled with Bacon	113
Rice and Vegetable Stuffed Tomatoes	114
Potato Halves with Bacon and Herbs	115
Cheese & Bacon Muffins	116
Asparagus Spears Rolled with Bacon	119
Fried Potatoes with Mushrooms	120
Potato Chips	122

Breaded Mushrooms	123
Brussels Sprout with Bacon	124
Poultry Recipes	126
Chicken with Spaghetti	126
Crispy Fried Wings	127
Breaded Chicken Tenders	129
Chicken Breasts with Cream Sauce	130
Sausage Stuffed in Chicken Fillet	131
Crispy Chicken Fillet with Cheese	132
Korean Chicken	133
Classic Crispy Chicken Wings	134
Chicken Tenders with Honey	135
Delicious Meat Recipes	137
Pork Chop	137
Rib Eye Steak	139
Fried Beef with Potatoes and Mushrooms	140
Pork Tenderloin	141
Meatballs Stewed in Yogurt	143
Cheese Stuffed Burgers	144
Fish & Seafood Recipes	146
Crab Pillows	146
Spring Rolls Stuffed with Shrimps	148
Yummy Shrimps with Bacon	150

Fried Crab Chips	150
Cod with Tomatoes	152
Salmon in Delicious Sauce	153
Tender Tuna Nuggets	154
Cod Pillows	156
Miso Tilapia	157
Potatoes with Garlic, Tomatoes and Shrimps	158
Dessert Recipes	160
Indian Banana Chips	160
Berry Pleasure	161
Fried Bananas with Ice Cream	162
Apple Wedges with Cinnamon	163
Fried Bananas	164
Pumpkin Cake	166
Conclusion	168

Part 1

Appetizers

Recipe #1 – Air Fried Onion Rings

Ingredients:

- 1 sweet onion, sliced thinly
- 1 teaspoon salt
- 1 teaspoon paprika
- 1/2 teaspoon garlic powder
- A bowl of ice water
- 1 cup self-rising flour

Directions:

1. Preheat the Air Fryer to 400°F.
2. Put ice water in a bowl. Soak the onion slices for 10 minutes.
3. In another bowl, mix to combine flour, paprika, salt, pepper, and garlic powder.
4. Get the onion slices using a pair of tongs. Put them in the bowl with the seasoned flour. Toss to coat and shake off the excess.
5. Layer each in the Air Fryer basket. Shake twice. Transfer to a plate and cook the rest of the onions. Serve.

Recipe #2 – Air-Fried Heart of Palms

Ingredients:
- 2 cans hearts of palm, halved lengthwise
- 1 cup panko breading
- 1 cup almond flour, finely milled
- 1 cup almond milk
- Pinch of salt
- Pinch of white pepper

Directions:
1. Preheat the Air Fryer to 330 degrees F.
2. Meanwhile, place flour, milk, and panko breading into 3 different shallow bowls. Dredge one heart of palms in flour first, and then into the milk; coat generously with panko breading.
3. Repeat step until all heart of palms are breaded. Place heart of palms in the Air Fryer basket. Fry these in oil until crisp and golden brown. Drain on paper towels.
4. Season with salt and pepper. Serve.

Recipe #3 – Air Fried Spinach Leaves

Ingredients:
- 1 pound fresh spinach leaves and tender stems
- Pinch, generous salt
- 1 cup almond flour, finely milled

Directions:
1. Preheat Air Fryer to 330 degrees F.
2. Season spinach leaves with salt. Dredge into flour.
3. Place breaded spinach leaves in the Air Fryer basket.
4. Fry until golden brown on both sides. Transfer cooked pieces on a plate lined with paper towels to remove excess grease.
5. Serve plain or with condiment of choice.

Recipe #4 - Cheese Sticks

Ingredients:
- 2 cups Italian seasoned breadcrumbs
- 2 eggs, beaten
- 1/4 cup grated Parmesan cheese

- 1/4 cup all-purpose flour
- 12 strings of part-skim mozzarella string cheese
- Marinara sauce for dipping or any dipping of choice

Directions:

1. Preheat Air Fryer to 400 degrees F.
2. Separate the cheese strings, arrange in a tray, and leave in the freezer for 2 hours.
3. Put parmesan cheese and breadcrumbs in a small bowl and mix until combined.
4. Crack and beat the eggs in another bowl. Put flour in a Ziploc bag.
5. Place the frozen cheese strings in the Ziploc bag with flour. Seal the bag and shake until all sides of the strings are coated. Dip each string in the bowl of beaten egg and coat with the breadcrumbs and cheese mixture.
6. Cook 6 cheese sticks for each batch. Place them in the cooking basket of the fryer and cook for 7 minutes.
7. Flip the cheese sticks and continue cooking for 3 minutes. Transfer to a plate and cook the rest of the cheese sticks.

Serve while warm along with the dipping sauce.

Recipe #5 – All Vegetable Fritters

Ingredients:
- ½ cup sweet potato, grated
- 1 cup squash, grated
- 1 shallot, peeled, minced
- 1 tsp. garlic powder
- ½ cup carrot, grated
- Pinch of salt
- Pinch of white pepper, to taste

Directions:
1. Preheat Air Fryer to 330 degrees F.
2. Combine ingredients into bowl. Mix well. Roll into 8 large balls or 12 smaller ones; flatten slightly.
3. Place vegetable fritters in the Air Fryer basket. Fry fritters until crisp and golden brown on all sides. Drain on paper towels. Serve.

Breakfast Recipes

Recipe #6 - Cheesy Ham and Egg in Potato Crust

Ingredients:

Fillings
- ¼ cup cooked ham , julienned
- ¼ tsp. red bell pepper, minced
- ½ tsp. chives, minced
- ¼ tsp. cheddar cheese, grated
- Pinch of sea salt
- Pinch of white pepper
- 2 eggs, whisked
- 1 Tbsp. fresh milk

Crust
- ½ cup potato, grated
- ⅛ tsp. olive oil, for greasing

Directions:

1. Preheat the Air Fryer to 400°F.
2. Grease ramekins using olive oil. Spread potatoes evenly into the ramekins.
3. Put ramekins in the Air Fryer basket. Cook for 5 minutes.
4. Remove ramekins and then flip potatoes. Do not remove ramekins just yet.
5. Reduce the heat of the Air Fryer to 330°F.
6. For the filling, scatter cooked ham on top of the potato crusts.
7. Meanwhile, put together red bell pepper, eggs, milk, chives, salt, pepper, cheddar cheese, and ham in a bowl. Whisk until all ingredients come together.
8. Pour mixture into ramekins. Place in the Air Fryer basket_again. Cook for 10 minutes or until set.
9. Remove ramekins from the Air Fryer. Transfer to a plate. Serve.

Recipe #7 – Air Fryer Hash Browns

Ingredients:
- 2 cups potatoes, diced
- ¼ cup chives, minced
- 3 cups water
- Olive oil

Directions:
1. Preheat the Air Fryer to 360°F. Prepare parchment paper. Cut out to 5x5.
2. Pour water into a saucepan. Drop potatoes. Season with salt. Bring mixture to a rolling boil.
3. The moment it boils, reduce the heat. Let simmer for 15 minutes.
4. Drain the potatoes and cool.
5. Mash potatoes using a large bowl. Stir in chives.
6. Shape mashed potato into thick patties. Make sure they are evenly shaped. Place each patty on a parchment paper.
7. Place patties into the Air Fryer basket. Put on the double layer rack into the Air Fryer. Cook 10 minutes or until golden brown.
8. Flip the other side and cook for another 3 minutes. This time without the parchment paper.

9. Remove from the Air Fryer. Transfer to a plate. Serve.

Recipe #8 - Air-Fried Spinach Eggs

Ingredients:

- 2 eggs
- 1 cup baby spinach
- 1/2 cup cheddar cheese, shredded
- Pinch of salt
- Pinch of pepper
- 4 slices Canadian bacon
- 1 tablespoon olive oil

Directions:

1. Preheat Air Fryer to 350 degrees F.
2. Cook spinach until wilted. Set aside.
3. Divide cooked spinach into greased ramekins.
4. Crack an egg on each ramekin. Scatter cheese and bacon top of each ramekin.
5. Place ramekins into the Air Fryer basket. Cook for 15 minutes. Serve.

Recipe #9 – Onion and Mushrooms Frittata

Ingredients:
- 4 eggs
- 1 red onion, sliced into thin rounds
- 4 cups button mushrooms, sliced thinly
- 4 tbsps. feta cheese, crumbled
- Pinch of salt
- 1 tbsp. olive oil

Directions:

1. Preheat Air Fryer to 330 degrees F.
2. Sauté onion rounds and button mushrooms in a pan set over medium heat. Transfer to a plate.
3. Meanwhile, whisk eggs in a bowl. Season with salt. Grease a baking dish with olive oil.

4. Pour egg mixture. Add in sautéed onions and mushroom. Sprinkle feta cheese on top.
5. Place baking dish into the Air Fryer basket. Cook for 20 minutes Serve.

Recipe #10 – Cheesy Sunny Side Up

Ingredients:

- 2 eggs, white and yolk separated
- ¼ cup mozzarella cheese, shredded
- ⅛ cup chives, minced
- Pinch of salt
- ⅛ tsp. olive oil

Directions
1. Preheat the Air Fryer to 360°F.
2. Lightly grease ramekins with olive oil.
3. Meanwhile, whisk the egg in a bowl, egg white first. Stir in half of the mozarella cheese and chives. Beat until all ingredients come together.
4. Pour mixture into a ramekin. Top with unbroken egg yolk.

5. Repeat the same step all over again for the remaining ingredients.
6. Place ramekins into the Air Fryer basket. Cook for 7 minutes or until are set.
7. Remove ramekins from the Air. Serve.

Recipe #11 – Carrots and Potatoes Frittata

Ingredients:

- 4 eggs
- 1 red onion, sliced thinly
- 1 small carrot, chopped
- 1 small potato, chopped
- 4 tablespoons feta cheese, crumbled
- 2 tablespoons olive oil
- Pinch of salt

Directions:

1. Preheat the pan in a stove. Pour olive oil. Saute onions, carrots, and potatoes for 3 minutes. Set aside.
2. Meanwhile, crack eggs in a bowl. Season with salt. Whisk well.

3. Pour whisked eggs on a greased baking dish. Scatter cooked onions, carrots and potatoes on top.
4. Place baking dish into the Air fryer basket. Cook for 30 minutes at 330 degrees F.

Recipe #12 - Tuna Cheese Sandwich
Ingredients:
- 1/2 cup sharp cheddar cheese, shredded
- 1 can solid white tuna in water, drained well
- 1/8 teaspoon celery salt
- 1 teaspoon onion, chopped finely
- Pinch black pepper
- 2 slices of bread
- 2 tablespoons mayonnaise
- 4 slices ripe tomato
- 1 celery stalk, chopped finely

Directions:

1. Preheat the Air Fryer to 400 degrees. Layer bread slices in the cooking basket. Cook for 3 minutes. Set aside.
2. Meanwhile, put together tuna, onion, celery, mayonnaise, salt, and pepper in a bowl. Mix well.
3. Spread mixture over slices of toasted bread slices.
4. Add 2 tomato slices and cheddar cheese on top.
5. Place one sandwich in Air Fryer cooking basket at a time. Cook for 4 minutes. Serve immediately.

Recipe #13 - Potatoes Gratin
Ingredients:
- 1/2 cup milk
- Pinch of ground black pepper
- 1/2 cup Gruyère cheese, grated
- 5 medium Russet potatoes, chopped into wafer-thin slices
- 1/2 cup cream

- 1/2 teaspoon Nutmeg

Directions:

1. Preheat Air Fryer to 390 degrees F.
2. Place potatoes in a bowl. Add in milk, nutmeg, cream, salt, and pepper.
3. Pour mixture into the potato. Make sure everything's coated.
4. Transfer potatoes into the baking dish. Place in the air fryer. Cook for 25 minutes.
5. Top with cheese. Cook for another 10 minutes or until the gratin is golden brown. Serve.

Recipe #14 - Scrambled Eggs On Toast

Ingredients:

Scrambled eggs

- 2 eggs, whisked until frothy
- 2 Tbsp. cream, chilled
- 1 tsp. cheddar cheese, grated
- 2 buffalo mozzarella, torn

- ⅛ lemon juice, freshly squeezed
- ⅛ tsp. olive oil, for greasing
- Pinch of black pepper, to taste

   For the Bread
- 2 wholegrain bread

- 2 ripe tomatoes, sliced, for garnish
- 1 cucumbers, sliced, for garnish
- Pinch of sea salt

   Directions
1. Preheat the Air Fryer to 360°F. Grease ramekins with olive oil.
2. In a bowl, whisk eggs, lemon juice, cheddar cheese, and cream.
3. Pour mixture over ramekins. Place into the Air Fryer basket. Cook for 10 minutes.
4. Once don, dot mozzarella cheese into the ramekins. Cook for another 5 minutes.
5. Remove from Air Fryer. Season with black pepper.

6. Meanwhile, place bread in the Air Fryer with the same heat. Cook for 2 minutes. Remove and set aside.
7. To serve, layer bread slice. Scoop just the right amount of scrambled eggs. Place tomatoes and cucumbers on top.

Recipe #15 – Cheesy Zucchini Omelet

Ingredients:
- 1 egg white
- 1 cooked zucchini, shredded
- Parmesan cheese, grated
- Olive oil, as needed
- Pinch of salt
- Pinch of pepper

Directions:
1. Preheat the Air Fryer to 330 degrees F.

2. Meanwhile, put together egg white, zucchini, cheese, salt, and pepper in a bowl.
3. Pour zucchini mixture into ramekins. Cook for 2 minutes on each side. Serve.

Recipe #16 - Tomato Leeks Frittata

Ingredients:

- 8 eggs
- 2 leeks, sliced
- 2 tomatoes
- 2 teaspoons olive oil
- ¼ cup milk
- ½ cup cheddar cheese
- 1 tablespoon fresh thyme
- Pinch of salt
- Pinch of pepper

Directions

1. Preheat the Air Fryer to 330 degrees F.
2. Lightly grease baking dish with olive oil. Add in eggs, leeks, cheese, salt, and pepper. Layer tomato slices on top.
3. Place into the Airfryer basket. Cook for 10 minutes.
4. Remove and transfer the frittata to a plate. Sprinkle with thyme before serving.

Recipe #17 – Golden Bacon Cheese Rolls
Ingredients:
Breading
- 2 eggs, beaten
- 1 cup all-purpose flour
- 1 cup Breadcrumbs, seasoned
- 4 tablespoons olive oil

Filling
- 1 lb. bacon slices
- 1 cup cheddar cheese, sliced into ¾-inch portions

Directions:
1. Preheat the Air Fryer at 390 degrees F.

2. Cover each piece of cheddar cheese with 2 bacon slices. Arrange on a tray. Place inside the freezer for 5 minutes.
3. Meanwhile, put together oil and breadcrumbs.
4. Dip each bacon-wrapped cheese in flour, on beaten eggs, and then onto the breadcrumbs.
5. Cook in the air fryer for about 7 minutes or until golden. Serve.

Recipe #18 - Feta Cheese Triangles
Ingredients:
- 4 ounces feta cheese
- 2 sheets frozen filo pastry, thawed
- 1 scallion, minced
- 2 tablespoons flat-leafed parsley, minced
- 1 egg yolk
- Pinch of ground black pepper
- 2 tablespoons olive oil

Directions:
1. Preheat the Air Fryer at 390 degrees F.

2. Put parsley, egg yolk, scallion, and feta in a bowl. Whisk for a couple of minutes and season with pepper.
3. Cut each filo sheet into 3 strips. Put 1 teaspoon of the yolk and feta mixture in every strip. Fold the tip of the sheet over the filling to form a triangle. Fold like a zigzag to wrap all filling.
4. Brush each filo with little oil. Cook 6 pieces for each batch. Arrange them in the cooking basket of the fryer and cook for 3 minutes.
5. Reduce temperature to 360 degrees and cook for 2 more minutes.

Recipe #19 - Fried Plantains with Coconut Almond Flakes

Ingredients:

- 4 ripe plantains, quartered lengthwise
- ¼ cup almond flakes, toasted
- ¼ cup coconut flakes, toasted

Directions:

1. Preheat Air Fryer to 330 degrees F.
2. Place plantains in the Air Fryer basket. Fry plantains until seared golden on both sides.

3. Garnish with almond and coconut flakes. Serve.

Recipe #20 - Potato Wedges
Ingredients:
- 2 potatoes, sliced into wedges
- 1 teaspoon dried thyme
- 1/2 tablespoon dried rosemary
- 1 teaspoon garlic powder
- 1 egg, beaten
- 1/4 cup grated parmesan cheese
- 1/2 teaspoon paprika
- Pinch of salt
- Pinch of pepper

Directions:
1. Preheat Air Fryer to 400 degrees F.
2. Mix parmesan, rosemary, garlic powder, salt, pepper, thyme, and paprika in a bowl.
3. Soak the potato wedges in the beaten egg and coat them with the cheese and spice mixture. Arrange in the cooking basket of the fryer.

4. Lightly spray with oil and cook for 20 minutes. Shake the basket twice during the cooking process.

Lunch Recipes

Recipe #21 Tuna Steaks with Spicy Cauliflower Pops

Ingredients:

For the cauliflower pops
- 1 head cauliflower, cut into bite-sized florets
- 2 Tbsp. olive oil
- Dash of cayenne powder
- Dash of curry powder
- Pinch of sea salt
- Pinch of white pepper

For the tuna steaks
- 2 bone-in tuna steaks
- 1 Tbsp. olive oil Pinch of salt

- 1 Tbsp. homemade garlic and parsley butter, for garnish
- 2 Tbsp. toasted garlic flakes, divided, for garnish

- ½ piece, small lemon, cut into wedges, for garnish

    Directions:
1. Preheat Air Fryer to 330 degrees F.
2. Put curry powder, cayenne powder, salt, and pepper in a paper bag. Seal bag and shake well together with cauliflower florets.
3. Place florets on the baking sheets. Drizzle olive oil on top. Put baking dish inside the Airfryer basket. Fry for 20 minutes or until cauliflower turns brown.. Set aside.
4. For the tuna steaks, season tuna with salt.
5. Layer tuna inside the Air Fryer basket. Fry for 2 minutes on each side. Transfer on a plate.
6. place steaks in each plate. Spread parsley and garlic butter. Add cauliflower pops. Serve with lemon wedges.

Recipe #22 - Shirataki Curry Noodle

Ingredients:
- 2 pounds shirataki noodles, packed in water
- 12 ounces tofu, extra firm
- 4 spring onions, chopped finely
- 12 pieces shrimp, cooked
- 1/2 teaspoon garlic powder
- 6 tablespoons Thai green curry paste
- 12 ounces napa cabbage
- 6 tablespoons soy sauce, divided
- 2 teaspoons lemongrass paste
- 1/4 pound mushrooms, sliced thinly
- 1 teaspoon sesame oil
- 1 red pepper, medium, sliced thinly
- 1 teaspoon coriander paste
- 1 ½ tablespoons fish sauce
- 3 tablespoons lime juice, freshly squeezed
- 4 tablespoons rice vinegar
- 5 ounces snow peas
- 1 piece green pepper, sliced thinly
- 1 cup water chestnuts, chopped
- 1 carrot, shredded

Directions:
1. Preheat Air Fryer to 320 degrees F.
2. Drain the noodles and rinse well before placing in a large bowl. Pour in boiling water as well as the soy sauce. Stir to coat the noodles on all sides.
3. In a small bowl, combine the soy sauce, sesame oil, garlic powder, and fish sauce.
4. Chop the tofu into half-inch cubes before adding to the sesame mixture. Toss until coated. Marinate for a few hours.
5. Mix the vegetables in a large bowl. Combine the lime juice, curry paste, coriander paste, lemongrass paste, and rice vinegar in another bowl. Arrange the cabbage, carrots, and spring onion on a platter.
6. Drain and spread the marinated tofu pieces on a plate. Mist with cooking spray before placing in the air fryer basket. Cook for about six minutes on each side or until crisp and golden. Transfer onto a plate covered with foil and set aside.
7. Add the shrimp to the air fryer basket. Coat with cooking spray and cook for two

to three minutes on each side. Set aside on a covered plate as well.
8. In a medium bowl, combine the tofu marinade with the rice vinegar, and curry paste. Pour into the air fryer basket. Add the vegetables and mist the mixture with cooking spray. Allow the veggies to cook for 5 minutes.
9. Place the drained noodles in a large bowl. Add the roasted veggies, tofu cubes, fresh veggies, and dressing. Toss to combine. Serve with shrimp.

Recipe #23 – Tomato Meatballs with Roasted Onions and Peppers
Ingredients:
- 1 egg
- 3/4 lbs. ground beef
- 1 onion
- 1 tablespoon fresh, parsley, chopped
- 1/2 tablespoon fresh thyme leaves, chopped
- 3 tablespoons panko breadcrumbs

- 1/2 cup tomato sauce
- 1/4 teaspoon salt
- 1/4 teaspoon pepper, freshly cracked

- 12 bell peppers
- 1 onion, chopped finely
- 1 tablespoon seasoning sauce
- 1 tablespoon olive oil

Directions:

1. Preheat the Air Fryer to 390 degrees F.
2. Place all ingredients in a bowl. Mix well until all ingredients come together. Mold into meatballs.
3. Place meatballs into the air fryer basket. Cook for 8 minutes. Transfer to a baking dish.
4. Pour tomato sauce all over. Return to the air fryer.
5. Cook meatballs for another 5 minutes at 330 degrees F. Set aside.
6. Meanwhile, pour olive oil into the baking dish. Add in onion, bell peppers, and seasoning sauce.

7. Mix well. Place into the air fryer to cook for 25 minutes. Pour mixture over meatballs. Serve.

Recipe #24 - Beef Tenderloin with Sautéed Onions and Peppers

Ingredients:

- 2½ lbs. beef tenderloin
- ½ red bell pepper, deseeded, ribbed, julienned
- 1 banana chili, julienned
- ½ green bell pepper, julienned
- 2 onions, julienned
- 2 tablespoons light soy sauce
- 1 cup almond flour, finely milled
- 3 tablespoons olive oil
- Pinch of palm sugar, crumbled
- Pinch of sea salt
- Pinch of black pepper

Directions:

1. Preheat the Air Fryer to 330 degrees F.
2. Place beef in a food-safe bag. Pour marinade ingredients. Shake and massage beef. Place inside the fridge for 1 hour or overnight.
3. Once done, place marinated beef in the Airfryer basket. Cook for 5 minutes on each side. Repeat the same cooking procedure as with the remaining meat.
4. Meanwhile, in a pan, saute onions and peppers for 2 minutes. Spoon in a plate. Serve with beef tenderloin.

Recipe #25 – Air Fried Beef Meatballs in Tomato Sauce

Ingredients:

- 3/4 pound ground beef
- 1 onion, chopped
- 1 tablespoon parsley, chopped
- 1 egg
- Pinch of salt

- Pinch of pepper
- 3 tablespoons breadcrumbs
- 1/2 tablespoon fresh thyme leaves, chopped
- 1 ½ cup tomato sauce

Directions:
1. Preheat the Air Fryer at 390 degrees F.
2. Mix all ingredients in a bowl. Shape them into balls of equal size
3. Layer in the Air Fryer basket. Cook for 8 minutes.
4. Transfer meatballs in an oven dish. Pour tomato sauce all over.
5. Place the oven dish in the Air Fryer basket. Cook for 5 minutes. Serve.

Recipe #26 – Country-Style Chicken
Ingredients:
For the breading
- 3 eggs, beaten
- 1 cup all-purpose flour

- 1 cup breadcrumbs
- 2 tbsp. olive oil
- 1/2 tsp. salt
- Pinch of black pepper, to taste

- 1 lb. chicken tenders

    Directions:

1. Preheat the Air Fryer to 330 degrees F.
2. Pour eggs and olive oil, breadcrumbs and salt, and then flour in three separate bowls.
3. Season with salt and pepper. Dredge chicken tenders into the flour. Dip in eggs, and then coat with breadcrumbs.
4. Place chicken tenders in the Air Fryer basket. Cook for 15 minutes. Serve.

Recipe #27 – Air Fried Asian Bok Choy

Ingredients:

- 3 cups chopped bok choy

- 1 garlic clove, minced
- 1 ½ tablespoon water
- ½ teaspoon honey
- 1 teaspoon light soy sauce
- 1 teaspoon cornstarch
- 1 tablespoon mirin
- 1 teaspoon olive oil

Directions:
1. Preheat the Air Fryer to 330 degrees F.
2. Put together honey, water, mirin, soy sauce, and cornstarch in a bowl. Pour into the saucepan. Bring to a boil. Transfer to a bowl. Set aside.
3. Meanwhile, place garlic and bok choy in the Air Fryer basket. Cook for 4 minutes. Transfer to a plate.
4. Pour sauce over vegetables. Serve.

Recipe #28 - Cajun-Style Shrimp
Ingredients:

- 1/2 lb. jumbo shrimp, peeled, deveined
- 1 egg
- 1/2 teaspoon garlic powder
- 1/4 teaspoon dried leaf thyme
- 1/4 teaspoon dried oregano
- 1 cup cornmeal
- 1 teaspoon cayenne pepper
- 1/2 cup all-purpose flour
- 1 teaspoon salt
- 1/8 teaspoon pepper

Directions:

1. Preheat the Air Fryer at 400 degrees F.
2. Put shrimp in a bowl and soak in cold water. Drain liquid and dry shrimp with paper towels.
3. Meanwhile, beat the eggs in another bowl. Add in cayenne, oregano, garlic powder, and thyme. Season with salt and black pepper. Mix well.
4. Spread flour in a plate and then the cornmeal in a separate plate.
5. Dredge shrimp in flour first, in the egg mixture. Coat with the cornmeal.

6. Layer shrimps in the Air Fryer basket. (Do not overcrowd Air Fryer. This can fit 6 shrimps) Cook for 10 minutes.

Recipe #29 - Chili Crab Legs

Ingredients:
- 2 lbs. frozen King crab legs, thawed, lightly drained
- 4 garlic clove, minced
- 1 Tbsp. butter
- ½ cup water
- ½ cup balsamic vinegar
- 2 banana chili, diced
- Pinch of fresh parsley
- Pinch of sea salt
- 1 Tbsp. olive oil

Directions:
1. Preheat the Air Fryer to 330 degrees F.
2. Pour olive oil, butter, and garlic in a pan. Saute garlic until golden brown.

3. Pour vinegar and water into the mixture. Season with salt and pepper. Bring to a boil.
4. Meanwhile, place crab legs into the Air Fryer basket. Cook for 5 minutes.
5. Transfer crab legs to the pan. Toss well until liquid is almost gone.
6. Garnish with banana chili and parsley. Serve.

Recipe #30 – Air Fried Baby Back Ribs
Ingredients:

- 1 slab baby back ribs
- 1 garlic clove, minced
- 1 teaspoon ginger, grated
- 1 jalapeño, chopped
- 1 scallion, finely chopped
- 1/2 tablespoon cilantro, chopped
- 1 cup orange juice
- 2 tablespoons sesame oil

Directions:

1. Preheat the Air Fryer to 350 degrees F.
2. Place all ingredients in a Ziploc bag. Seal and massage. Leave for 1 hour or overnight in the fridge to marinate. Reserve marinade sauce.
3. Place baby back ribs in the Air Fryer basket in a vertical position. Cook for 35 minutes.
4. Meanwhile, pour marinade liquid in a pan. Cook until the liquid is reduced by half.
5. Brush the half-cooked ribs with the marinade. Continue cooking for 30 minutes.
6. Slice meat before serving along with the remaining marinade sauce. Serve.

Recipe #31 – Citrusy Buttered Tilapia

Ingredients:

- 2 large tilapia fillets, skin-on
- 2 tsp. Spanish paprika powder
- 1 tsp. sea salt
- 2 Tbsp. citrusy butter
- 1 Tbsp. fresh cilantro, minced

Directions:
1. Preheat the Air Fryer to 330 degrees F.
2. Season tilapia with paprika and salt. Let drain in a colander for 20-30 minutes.
3. Place tilapia in the Air Fryer basket. Fry fillets for 5 minutes or until crisp tender and brown all over.
4. Transfer to a plate. Pour citrusy butter. Garnish with cilantro. Serve.

Recipe #32 - Chicken Fries with Grilled Tomatoes

Ingredients:
- 4 chicken legs, skin on
- 1 tablespoon garlic powder
- 1 tablespoon Paprika
- 1 teaspoon onion powder
- 1/2 teaspoon poultry seasoning
- 1 teaspoon cumin
- 1 tablespoon olive oil
- 3 pieces chicken thighs, skin on
- 1 cup whole buttermilk

- 1 tablespoon ground black pepper
- 2 cups white flour

- 2 tomatoes, halved
- 1/4 teaspoon pepper
- 1/4 teaspoon mixed herbs

Directions:

1. Preheat the Air Fryer to 320 degrees F. Sprinkle mixed herbs and pepper on tomatoes. Layer on the Air Fryer basket. Cook for 20 minutes.
2. Meanwhile, place chicken in a bowl. Add in buttermilk. Mix well. Place inside the fridge to marinate for 1-2 hours.
3. In another bowl, put together flour with the seasonings. Remove chicken from the fridge.
4. Coat chicken pieces with the flour mixture. Dip in the buttermilk mixture and then to the flour mixture again.
5. Layer coated chicken in the Air Fryer basket. Drizzle in olive oil. Cook for 20 minutes. Turn chicken every 5 minutes.
6. Serve with the roasted tomatoes.

Recipe #33 - Chicken Skewer

Ingredients:

- 12 ounces chicken tenders
- 1 tablespoon ginger, grated
- 4 garlic cloves, chopped
- 4 scallions, chopped
- 2 teaspoons toasted sesame seeds
- 1/2 cup pineapple juice
- 1/2 cup low-sodium soy sauce
- 1/4 cup sesame oil
- A pinch of black pepper

Directions:

1. Preheat the Air Fryer to 390 degrees F.
2. Place meat on a skewer.
3. Pour the rest of the ingredients in a bowl. Mix well. Marinate skewered meat on the prepared mixture.
4. Place inside the fridge for 2 hours or overnight.

5. Pat the meat dry with paper towels. Layer skewered meat in the Air Fryer basket. Cook for 7 minutes. Serve.

Recipe #34 – Air Fried Pork Tenderloin

Ingredients:
- 2 pork tenderloin, sliced into matchsticks
- 1 white onion, sliced thinly
- ½ red bell pepper, julienned
- ½ green bell pepper, julienned
- 1 Tbsp. almond flour, finely milled
- 1 Tbsp. cooking oil
- 1 tsp. sea salt
- 1 tsp. ground black pepper

Directions:
1. Preheat the Air Fryer to 330 degrees F.
2. Season pork tenderloin with pepper flakes, salt, pepper, and almond flour. Set aside.

3. Place into the Air Fryer basket. Cook for 5 minutes.
4. Meanwhile, heat oil in a pan. Stir fry onions and bell peppers.
5. Serve air fried pork in a plate with onions and bell peppers on the side.

Bonus Lunch Recipes

Moroccan Meatballs with Mint Yogurt
Ingredients:
- 1 pound ground lamb
- 4 ounces ground turkey
- 1 egg white
- 1 teaspoon red chili paste
- 2 garlic cloves, minced
- 1 teaspoon cayenne pepper
- 1 1/2 tablespoons chopped parsley
- 1 tablespoon mint, chopped
- 1 teaspoon ground coriander
- 1 teaspoon salt
- 1 teaspoon ground cumin
- 1/4 cup olive oil

For the mint yogurt
- 1/2 cup Greek yogurt
- 1 garlic clove, minced
- 2 tablespoons buttermilk
- 1/4 cup chopped mint
- 1/4 cup sour cream
- Pinch of salt

Directions:
1. Preheat the Air Fryer to 390 degrees F.
2. Put all ingredients for the meatballs in a bowl. Mix until combined. Divide the mixture and roll each into a golf-size ball. Arrange the pieces in the cooking basket of the fryer. Cook for 8 minutes.
3. Prepare the mint yogurt. Put all the ingredients in a bowl and mix well. Season with salt. Top with olives and fresh mint.
4. Transfer the cooked meatballs on a plate and serve along with the sauce.

Crusted Lamb
Ingredients:
- 1 ¾ pounds lamb rack
- 1 garlic clove
- 1 tablespoon olive oil
- 1/4 teaspoon salt
- 1/4 teaspoon pepper

Crust
- 3 oz macadamia nuts, unsalted
- 1 egg
- 1 tablespoon panko breadcrumbs
- 1 tablespoon fresh rosemary, chopped

Directions:
1. Preheat the Air Fryer at 220 degrees F.
2. Chop the garlic into fine bits and mix with the olive oil. Brush this mixture on the lamb before sprinkling with salt and pepper.
3. After chopping the macadamia nuts into bits, add to a bowl filled with the rosemary and breadcrumbs. Stir to combine.
4. Whisk the egg in a deep dish and set aside.
5. Dip the lamb into the whisked egg before coating with the macadamia mixture.

6. Place in the air fryer and cook for thirty minutes. Increase heat to 390 degrees F. cook for a 5 minutes.
7. Transfer the lamb to a plate. Cover with foil and let sit for ten minutes. Serve.

Creamy Chicken Mushrooms

Ingredients

- 4 chicken thigh fillets, cubed
- 1 can thick coconut cream
- ½ Tbsp. ginger, grated
- 1 bird's eye chili, minced
- 1 Tbsp. lemongrass bulb, minced
- Pinch of sea salt, add more if needed
- Pinch of white pepper, to taste
- 1½ cups rice, cooked
- ⅛ cup cilantro, minced
- 1 can button mushrooms, quartered

Directions:

1. Preheat the Air Fryer to 355 degrees F.

2. For the chicken, combine chicken thigh fillets, coconut cream, ginger, bird's eye chili, lemongrass bulb, salt, and pepper in a mixing bowl. Mix well. Place inside the fridge for 1 hour.
3. Meanwhile, spread cooked rice into the tiffin box. Scatter button mushrooms on top.
4. Pour marinade sauce over the rice and mushrooms. Seal and secure the lid of the tiffin box. Allow marinade sauce to seep through the rice and mushrooms.
5. Place tiffin box into the Air Fryer basket. Cook for 5 minutes.
6. Reduce the heat to 285 degrees °F. Cook for another 15 minutes. Turn off the machine. Let the tiffin box cool for a few minutes before removing from the basket.
7. Garnish with cilantro. Serve and eat right out of tiffin box.

Mushroom Chickpea Burger

Ingredients:
- 2 hamburger buns, halved, toasted
- ½ tsp. pesto
- 2 slices tomatoes
- ½ cup mozzarella cheese, shredded

For the Veggie Patty
- 1 can chickpeas
- 2 sun-dried tomatoes in olive oil, lightly drained
- 2 Tbsp. pine nuts, roasted, shelled, lightly salted
- 1 can button mushrooms
- 1/16 tsp. garlic powder
- ⅛ tsp. Italian seasonings
- 1/16 tsp. black pepper
- ⅛ tsp. olive oil, add more if needed
- ½ tsp. oats, add more if needed
- ¼ cup fresh chives, minced

Directions:
1. Preheat the Air Fryer to 355°F.
2. Lightly grease two ramekins with oil.
3. Using a food processor, put together chickpeas, tomatoes, pine nuts, button

mushrooms, garlic powder, Italian seasonings, and black pepper. Process until just combined.
4. Transfer mixture over a bowl. Add in oats and chives.
5. Pour equal amounts of the mixture into the ramekins. Put the ramekins into the Air Fryer basket. Cook for 10 minutes.
6. Dot each patty with mozzarella cheese. Cook for another 5 minutes.
7. To serve, spread pesto on the hamburger buns. Top with veggie patties, tomato slice, and then the seal with the top bun.

Dinner Recipes

Recipe #35 – Air Fried Homemade Chicken Nuggets

Ingredients:

- 1 lb. chicken breasts, chopped
- 1/2 teaspoon garlic powder
- 1/2 teaspoon paprika
- 1 teaspoon salt
- 1 cup buttermilk
- 1 cup all-purpose flour

Directions:

1. Preheat the Air Fryer to 330 degrees F.
2. Put buttermilk in a bowl. Soak meat and leave to marinate for an hour or overnight.
3. Put flour, garlic powder, paprika, and salt in a bowl. Mix until combined. Add the marinated meat and toss to coat.
4. Place chicken nuggets in the air fryer basket. Cook for 10 minutes. Transfer to a plate. Cook the remaining nuggets. Serve.

Recipe #36 - Steak with Sausage Gravy and Potatoes

Ingredients:

- 6 ounces sirloin steak, pounded
- 6 ounces ground sausage meat
- 3 eggs, beaten
- 1 teaspoon pepper
- 1 teaspoon garlic powder
- 2 tablespoon flour
- 1 cup panko breadcrumbs
- 2 cups milk
- 1 cup flour
- 1 teaspoon onion powder
- 1 teaspoon salt

Roasted potatoes

- 2 lbs. potatoes, cubed
- 1 teaspoon olive oil

Directions:

1. Preheat the Air Fryer to 320 degrees F.
2. Heat a nonstick skillet. Cook sausage. Drain grease, but leave two tablespoons in the skillet.

3. Add in flour, then stream in milk. Cook until mixture is thickened. Season with pepper. cook for another 3 minutes. Set aside.
4. Place potato cubes in a bowl. Add in oil. Toss well to coat.
5. Place in the Air Fryer basket. Cook for 25 minutes.
6. Place the potatoes back in the bowl, toss, and load back in the air fryer. Cook for another 7 minutes more.
7. Meanwhile, put together spices with breadcrumbs. Coat steak in the flour, egg, and then the seasoned breadcrumbs.
8. Add coated steak to the air fryer basket. Cook for 12 minutes at 370 degrees F.
9. Pour gravy over steak. Serve with potatoes.

Recipe #37 - Beef Curry on Bed of Rice and Veggies

Ingredients:

For the Beef curry and sauce
- ½ beef tenderloin, sliced into strips
- Pinch of sea salt, add more if needed
- Pinch of white pepper
- ½ tsp. curry powder
- ⅛ tsp. ginger, grated
- Pinch of red pepper flakes
- 1 can thick coconut cream
- ½ tsp. garam masala
- ¼ tsp. ghee
- 1/16 tsp. fish sauce

- 1 cup brown rice, cooked

For the Veggies and Mushrooms
- 1 cup straw mushrooms, halved
- ¼ cup baby peas
- ¼ cup onions, diced
- ¼ cup cauliflower, sliced into bite-sized florets

Directions:
1. Preheat the Air Fryer to 355°F.
2. Season tenderloin with salt and pepper.

3. Meanwhile, in a mixing bowl, combine ginger, garam masala, curry powder, ghee, red pepper flakes, coconut cream, and fish sauce.
4. Spread cooked rice in a tiffin box. Scatter onions, baby peas, mushrooms, and cauliflower all over. Place beef slices on top of the vegetables.
5. Pour beef curry sauce over the tiffin box.
6. Place tiffin box into the Air Fryer basket. Cook for 5 minutes.
7. Cook for another 15 minutes with a reduced heat of 285°F.
8. Turn off machine. Leave tiffin box to rest inside for a few minutes. Serve.

Recipe #38 – Fried Salmon Fillets with Kale Chips

Ingredients:

Kale chips

- 1 pound fresh kale leaves, leaves snipped into squares
- 2 Tbsp. olive oil
- Pinch of sea salt

Salmon fillets
- <u>2 pieces salmon fillets</u>
- <u>¼ cup Parmigiano-Reggiano cheese, grated</u>
- <u>½ cup sour cream</u>
- <u>¼ cup cottage cheese</u>

- <u>Spanish paprika</u>

Directions:
1. Preheat Air Fryer to 330 degrees F.
2. Place kale leaves on a baking sheet. Season with salt. Drizzle in olive oil on top.
3. Put baking dish inside the Air Fryer basket. Cook for 15 minutes or until golden brown. Transfer to a plate. Set aside.
4. Mix Parmigiano-Reggiano cheese, sour cream, and cottage cheese in a bowl.
5. Layer salmon fillets in the Air Fryer basket. Cook for 20 minutes.

6. Place a salmon fillet and sprinkle paprika. Spread kale chips all over the fillet. Squeeze lemon juice all over. Serve.

Recipe #39 – Pepperoni Pizza Rolls
Ingredients:

- 10 egg roll wrappers
- 1 onion, chopped
- 2 red peppers, chopped
- 10 pepperoni slices, chopped
- 2 Italian sausage, cooked, crumbled
- 1 teaspoon garlic powder
- 2 cups mozzarella, shredded
- 1 14-ounce jar pizza sauce

Directions:

1. Preheat Air Fryer to 400 degrees F.
2. Put cheese, peppers, onions, pepperoni, and sausage in a bowl. Mix. Scoop 1/4 of the mixture into an egg roll wrapper.
3. Fold the sides of the wrapper. Secure the filling inside by putting a bit of water in the last fold. Leave in the freezer overnight.
4. Arrange rolls in the Air Fryer basket. Cook by batches for 7 minutes

5. Flip the pizza rolls and continue cooking for 2 minutes. Transfer to a plate and cook the rest of the rolls.
6. Serve with pizza sauce for dipping.

Recipe #40 – Air Fried Pork and Potatoes
Ingredients:

- 2 red potatoes, diced
- 1/2 teaspoon red pepper flakes
- 1 teaspoon pepper
- 1 tablespoon balsamic glaze
- 2 pounds pork loin
- 1 teaspoon salt
- 1/2 teaspoon garlic powder
- 1 teaspoon parsley

Directions:

1. Preheat Air Fryer to 390 degrees F.
2. Rub the seasonings all over the potatoes and pork loin.
3. Arrange the potatoes and pork in the Air Fryer basket. Cook for 25 minutes.
4. Transfer roasted pork and potatoes on a plate. Chop pork into slices. Drizzle in the balsamic glaze. Serve.

Recipe #41 – Air Fried Beef Dumplings

Ingredients:
- 12 circular pot sticker wrappers, separated

Filling
- ½ cup ground beef
- ⅛ tsp. ginger, grated
- ¼ cup napa cabbage, julienned
- ¼ Tbsp. green onions, minced
- ¼ tsp. miso paste
- 1 garlic clove, grated
- 1/16 tsp. white sugar
- ¼ tsp. sesame oil
- Pinch of sea salt

Dipping sauce
- 2 Tbsp. dark soy sauce
- 1 Tbsp. rice vinegar
- 1/16 tsp. chili oil

Directions
1. Preheat the Air Fryer to 400°F.

2. For the dumplings, put together ground beef, green onions, garlic clove, ginger, white sugar, miso paste, napa cabbage, sesame oil, and salt in a bowl. Mix until all ingredients are well combined.
3. Scoop an equal amount of the filled and place on the pot sticker.
4. Fold the wrapper into two. Seal the edges with water. Moisten the edges of the wrapper with water.
5. Repeat the same procedure until all pot stickers are used up. Layer on a baking sheet. Place inside the fridge for 1 hour. Freeze for an hour before frying.
6. Place frozen pot stickers into the Air Fryer basket. Do not overlap.
7. Cook for 10 minutes or until golden brown.
8. For the dipping sauce, combine rice wine vinegar, soy sauce, and chili oil in a mixing bowl. Set aside.
9. Serve with dipping sauce.

Recipe #42 - Chicken with Cauliflower
Ingredients:

For the quick fry
- 2 Tbsp. olive oil
- 1 garlic clove, minced
- 1 ginger, grated
- 2 stalks leeks, minced
- 1 can water chestnuts, quartered
- 1 cauliflower head, cut into bite-sized florets
- 1 red bell pepper, julienned
- ¾ cups chicken broth
- 1½ pounds chicken thigh fillets, diced

Seasonings
- Pinch of salt
- Pinch of black pepper, to taste
- ½ Tbsp. cornstarch, dissolved in
- 4 Tbsp. water
- 1 tsp. stevia
- 1 Tbsp. fish sauce

- leeks, minced
- 1 lime, cut into wedges

- 1½ cups cooked wild rice

Directions:
1. Preheat the Air Fryer to 330 degrees F.
2. Pour olive oil in a pan. Swirl pan to coat. Saute garlic, ginger, and leeks for 2 minutes. Set aside.
3. Add in water chestnuts, cauliflower, red bell pepper, and chicken broth. Stir well. Cook for 15 minutes.
4. Meanwhile, put the chicken in the Airfryer basket. Fry until seared and golden brown.
5. Add in seasoning into the pan. Stir and cook until the juice thickens.
6. Place cooked rice on the side of the plate. Ladle chicken and veggies.
7. Garnish with leeks and lemon wedges on the side. Serve.

Recipe #43 – Air Fried Coconut Shrimp
Ingredients:

- 1/2 pound jumbo shrimp
- 2 eggs
- 1/2 cup sweetened coconut flakes
- 1/2 cup cornstarch
- 1 tablespoon water
- 1/2 teaspoon salt
- 1/3 cup panko breadcrumbs

Directions:

1. Preheat the Air Fryer to 400 degrees F.
2. Place egg and water in a shallow baking dish. Beat until combined.
3. In another baking dish, put the coconut flakes, breadcrumbs, and salt. Mix well.
4. Put shrimp and cornstarch in a Ziploc bag. Seal and shake to coat.
5. Dip each shrimp in the egg mixture and then breadcrumb mixture.
6. Cook for 6 minutes. Transfer to a plate. Serve.

Recipe #44 - Turkey with Basil Pesto Tomatoes

Ingredients:

- 8 pounds turkey breast, skin on
- 2 tablespoons sea salt
- 1 tablespoon ground black pepper
- 2 tablespoons olive oil

Tomatoes

- 2 heirloom tomatoes, sliced into thick rounds
- 8 ounces feta cheese, sliced into half-inch thick rounds
- 1/2 cup red onions, sliced thinly
- 1 tablespoon olive oil
- Pinch of salt

Basil pesto

- 1/2 cup basil, chopped
- 1/2 cup parsley, chopped
- 1 garlic clove
- 3 tablespoons pine nuts, toasted
- 1/2 cup olive oil
- 1/2 cup parmesan cheese, shredded
- Pinch of salt

Directions:

1. Preheat the Air Fryer to 390 degrees F.
2. Fill the blender with the Parmesan, pine nuts, parsley, salt, garlic, and basil. Process while streaming in the olive oil. Set aside in the refrigerator.
3. Drizzle in olive oil into the red onions. Top with the pesto, feta cheese, and red onions. Place in the Air Fryer. Cook for 12 minutes. Set aside.
4. Brush olive oil all over turkey. Sprinkle seasonings. Add turkey to the air fryer and cook at 360 degrees for 20 minutes.
5. Turn the turkey to the other side and cook for another twenty minutes. Once done, let the turkey sit on a platter for twenty minutes. Serve with the basil pesto tomatoes.

Recipe #45 – Air Fried Aubergines and Tomatoes

Ingredients:
- 1 aubergine, sliced thickly into 4 disks

- 1 firm tomato, sliced thickly into 2 thick disks
- 2 fresh basil leaves, minced
- 2 balls buffalo mozzarella, torn
- 2 tsp. feta cheese
- Pinch of salt
- Pinch of black pepper

Directions:

1. Preheat Air Fryer to 330 degrees F.
2. Place aubergine slices into the Air Fryer basket. Cook for 5 minutes. Transfer to a plate.
3. Fry tomato slices in batches for 5 minutes or until seared on both sides.
4. To serve, stack salad starting with an aubergine base, buffalo mozzarella, basil leaves, tomato slice, and ½ teaspoon feta cheese.
5. Top of with another slice of aubergine and ½ tsp feta cheese. Serve.

Recipe #46 - Stuffed Garlic Mushrooms
Ingredients:

- 12 button mushrooms
  Stuffing
- 1 garlic clove, crushed
- 1 1/2 slices of white bread
- 1 tablespoon flat-leafed parsley, minced
- 1 1/2 tablespoons olive oil
- Ground black pepper

Directions:

1. Preheat the Air Fryer to 390 degrees F.
2. Put all bread slices in a food processor and process into fine crumbs. Add garlic, pepper, and parsley. Process until combined. Put in a bowl, add olive oil, and mix well.
3. Chop off the stalks of the mushrooms. Add breadcrumbs to their caps and pat them to stick. Cook for 8 minutes. Serve.

Bonus Recipes

Shrimps with Vegetables Roast

Ingredients:

- 12 large shrimps
- 1 cup dried coconut, unsweetened
- 1 cup egg white
- 1 tablespoon cornstarch
- 1 cup white flour
- 1 cup panko breadcrumbs

Vegetables

- 1 1/3 cups butternut squash, cubed
- 2 red onions, chopped into wedges
- 1 1/3 cups celery, cubed
- 1 tablespoon fresh thyme needles
- 1 1/3 cups parsnips, cubed
- 1 tablespoon olive oil
- 1/4 teaspoon salt
- 1/4 teaspoon pepper
- 2 tablespoons olive oil

Directions:

1. Preheat the Air Fryer to 350 degrees F.
2. Let the shrimps drain on a plate lined with paper towels.

3. Meanwhile, combine the coconut and breadcrumbs in a medium bowl. In a separate bowl, combine the cornstarch and flour as well.
4. Fill a small bowl with the egg white. Set aside.
5. Coat each shrimp with the flour mixture before dipping into the egg white. Coat with the coconut mixture and place in the air fryer basket.
6. Cook coated shrimp for 5 minutes before flipping on the other side. Cook for another 5 minutes. set aside.
7. Reset the air fryer at 390 degrees Fahrenheit.
8. Place all vegetables in a medium bowl. Add the salt, pepper, thyme, and olive oil. Toss to combine before loading into the air fryer basket. Cook for 10 minutes. Serve.

Bonus Recipe - Almond-Crusted Chicken Slivers

Ingredients:

- 3 large eggs, whisked
- 3 cups almond flour, coarsely milled
- ¼ cup almond slivers
- 1 lime, sliced into wedges, for garnish
- 1 cup all-purpose flour

Dip

- 1 tsp. honey
- ¼ cup Dijon mustard
- 2 Tbsp. mayonnaise
- Pinch of sea salt
- Pinch of black pepper

Chicken and dry rub

- 2 pounds chicken breast fillets, sliced into ½ inch thick slivers
- ½ tsp. ginger powder
- 1 tsp. garlic powder
- ½ tsp. cayenne pepper
- 1 tsp. white pepper
- ¼ tsp. brown sugar

- Dash of red pepper flakes

Directions:
1. Preheat Air Fryer to 330 degrees F.
2. Line 2 baking sheets with aluminum foil; lightly grease with oil. Set aside. Mix dip ingredients in a small bowl. Taste; adjust seasoning if needed.
3. Mix chicken and dry rub ingredients in bowl; marinate for 5 minutes.
4. Dredge chicken eat one piece at a time first in all-purpose flour, then in whisked egg, and finally in almond flour. Place on prepared baking sheet, making sure there are spaces in between. Top off with light sprinkling of almond slivers; cover loosely with aluminum foil.
5. Put baking sheet inside the Air Fryer basket. Fry for 25 minutes. Remove baking sheets; let chicken fingers cool for 5 minutes.
6. Serve equal portions of chicken fingers into plates; serve with dip and wedge of lime on the side. Squeeze lime juice over chicken fingers just before eating

Teriyaki Fish Steak

Ingredients:

- 1 lb. halibut steak
- 1/4 tsp. ground ginger
- 1 garlic clove, crushed
- 1/2 cup mirin
- ¼ cup sugar
- 2 tbsp. lime juice
- 1/4 cup orange juice
- 2/3 cup soy sauce
- 1/4 tsp. red pepper flakes, crushed

Directions:

1. Preheat the Air Fryer to 390 degrees F.
2. Combine garlic clove, mirin, ground cumin, lime juice, orange juice, sugar, soy sauce, and red pepper flakes in a saucepan. Bring mixture to a boil. Remove from heat and let cool.
3. Dredge the halibut steak on the marinade. Place inside a Ziploc bag. Seal and inside the fridge for 2 hours.

4. Once ready to cook, place the halibut steak in the Air Fryer basket. Cook for 12 minutes.
5. Brush the remaining marinade over the cooked halibut steaks. Serve.

Snacks and Desserts

Recipe #47 –Zucchini Rolls

Ingredients:

Cream cheese mix
- 1 tsp. sour cream
- ¼ cup cream cheese
- ⅛ cup fresh chives, minced
- Pinch of sea salt
- Pinch of white pepper

- 2 zucchini, shaved off into long slivers
- ¼ pound ham, sliced thinly

Directions:
1. Preheat the Air Fryer to 330 degrees F.
2. Combine sour cream, cream cheese, chives, salt, and pepper in a bowl to make the cream cheese mix.
3. Layer zucchini slivers in the Air Fryer basket. Spread cream cheese. Place ham on top and roll into bundles. Secure with a toothpick.
4. Cook for 4 minutes. Serve.

Recipe #48 - Doughnuts with Glaze

Ingredients:

- 1 can refrigerated croissant dinner rolls, sliced into rounds
- 1 can of vanilla frosting

Directions:

1. Preheat the Air Fryer to 400 degrees F.

2. Shape rounded croissant into a doughnut by tearing a hole in the middle. Do it with rest of the croissant rolls.
3. Place doughnuts in the Air Fryer basket. Cook for 2 minutes. Flip the other side and continue cooking for 3 more minutes. Do not overcrowd. Cook the remaining doughnuts.
4. For the frosting, place half a cup of the frosting in a bowl. Microwave for 30 seconds. Roll cooked doughnuts into the melted frosting. Leave for a couple of minutes until set. Serve.

Recipe #49 – Air Fried Chocolate Cake with Apricot Jam

Ingredients:

- 1 cup pure chocolate pieces
- 1 egg
- 1 tablespoon cocoa powder
- ½ cup apricot jam
- 1 cup flour

- 1 block butter
- 1 cup fine granulated sugar
- pinch of salt
- 1 teaspoon orange peel, grated

Directions:

1. Preheat the Air Fryer at 320 degrees F.
2. Place the sugar and butter in a medium bowl. Beat with a hand mixer until creamy and light.
3. Crack in egg. Beat until well-combined with the butter-sugar mixture. Stir in the cocoa powder, salt, and flour.
4. Add the grated orange peel, pure chocolate pieces, and apricot jam. Stir to combine and then pour into the greased cake pan. After smoothing the batter's surface with a spatula, place in the air fryer.
5. Cook for 25 minutes or until firm. Allow to cool for about five minutes before taking it out of the pan. Slice. Serve.

Recipe #50 - Apricot and Blueberries Crumble

Ingredients:

- 1 cup fresh apricots, cubed
- 1 cup fresh blackberries
- 1/2 cup sugar
- 1 cup flour
- Pinch of salt
- 2 tablespoons lemon juice
- 5 tablespoons cold butter

Directions:

1. Preheat the Air Fryer at 390 degrees F.
2. Put the blackberries, apricots, lemon juice, and 2 tablespoons of sugar in a bowl. Mix well and transfer to a baking dish.
3. In another bowl, put the remaining sugar, flour, and a pinch of salt. Mix until combined. Add 1 tablespoon of cold butter.
4. Rub the mixture using your hands until it becomes crumbly. Transfer to the baking dish on top of the fruit mixture and lightly press to compress.

5. Place the baking dish in the Air Fryer basket. cook for 20 minutes. Serve.

Recipe #51 - Mushroom Chicken Spring Rolls

Ingredients:

Filling

- 4 oz chicken breast, shredded, cooked
- 1 carrot, thinly sliced
- 1/2 teaspoon ginger, finely chopped
- 1/2 cup mushrooms, sliced thinly
- 1 stalk celery, sliced thinly
- 1 teaspoon chicken stock powder
- 1 teaspoon sugar

- 8 spring roll wrappers
- 1 egg, beaten
- 1 teaspoon cornstarch
- 1/2 teaspoon coconut oil

Directions:

1. Preheat the Air Fryer at 390 degrees F.
2. In a large bowl, combine the shredded chicken with the mushrooms, carrot, and celery. Stir in the chicken stock powder, ginger, and sugar.

3. Stir the cornstarch and egg together to form a paste.
4. Stuff the spring roll wrappers with divided portions of the chicken-mushroom filling. Brush the ends with the egg mixture. Seal by pinching.
5. Layer rolls into the Air Fryer basket. Cook for 4 minutes. Serve.

Recipe #52 – Raspberry Choco Cake

Ingredients:
- 2 eggs, whisked until frothy
- ½ cup all-purpose flour, sifted twice
- 2 Tbsp. powdered sugar, divided
- 1 cup dark chocolate buttons, melted
- ½ cup butter, divided
- 1 tsp. baking powder
- 1/16 tsp. vanilla essence
- ¼ lb. raspberries, for garnish

Directions:

1. Preheat the Air Fryer to 285°F.
2. Lightly grease aluminum muffin tins.
3. Put together eggs, butter, all-purpose flour, baking powder, melted dark chocolate, and vanilla essence in a mixing bowl. Whisk well.
4. Half fill muffin tins with the mixture. Place the tins in one layer into the Air Fryer basket.
5. Cook for 10 minutes. Remove from the basket. Loosen cake edges. Turn cake out into a dessert plate.
6. Top raspberries on cakes. Sprinkle powdered sugar. Serve.

Recipe #53 - Pepperoni Patties
Ingredients:
- 18 pieces pepperoni slices
- 1 lb. mozzarella
- 2 cups Italian breadcrumbs
- 4 egg, beaten

Directions:
1. Preheat the Air Fryer to 400°F.

2. Cut the mozzarella block into quarter-inch thick portions, then slice each piece in two.
3. Top each mozzarella piece with 2 pepperoni slices. Add the remaining mozzarella pieces to form cheese sandwiches.
4. Coat each cheese sandwich in flour before dipping into the eggs. Cover in breadcrumbs and mist with cooking spray.
5. Place in the air fryer. Cook for 3 minutes on each side. Serve.

Recipe #54 - Raspberry Cheesecake Rolls

Ingredients:

- 10 egg roll wrappers
- 2 1/2 cups cheesecake filling
- 1/4 cup white chocolate chips
- Powdered sugar for dusting
- 1 pint fresh raspberries

Directions:

1. Preheat the Air Fryer to 400°F.
2. Place the egg roll wrapper on a cutting board. Put 1/4 cup of the cheesecake filling at the center and top with 5 raspberries. Sprinkle with white chocolate chips.
3. Fold the wrapper over the filling, moisten the edges of the wrapper to seal, and roll tightly. Perform the steps until you're done with all the egg roll wrappers.
4. Cook 5 cheesecake rolls for each batch. Arrange them in the cooking basket of the fryer, lightly spray with oil, and cook for 7 minutes.
5. Flip the cheesecake rolls and continue cooking for 2 minutes. Transfer to a plate and cook the rest of the rolls.
6. Sprinkle rolls with powdered sugar before serving.

Recipe #55 – Air Fried Cheesy and Meaty Potato Skins

Ingredients:

- 2 Yukon Gold potatoes
- 2 green onions, minced
- 4 bacon strips
- 1/4 cup cheddar cheese, shredded
- 1/3 cup sour cream
- 1/4 teaspoon sea salt
- 1/2 teaspoon olive oil

Directions:
1. Preheat the Air Fryer to 400°F.
2. Rinse the potatoes in running water and scrub until clean. Rub with oil and season with salt.
3. Arrange them in the cooking basket of the fryer and cook for 35 minutes at 400 degrees. Transfer to a plate.
4. Arrange the bacon strips in the basket of the fryer and cook for 5 minutes at 400 degrees. Transfer to a bowl. Allow to cool and crumble into bits.
5. Slice each potato in half and scoop out most of the meat. Place the potato skins in the cooking basket with the skin side facing up. Cook for 3 minutes.

6. Turn them over and fill with cheese and crumbled bacon. Continue cooking for 2 minutes.
7. Transfer to a plate. Top each with sour cream and onion. Serve.

Recipe #56 – Air Fried Pork Cracklings

Ingredients:
- 1½ pounds whole pork rind, scored thrice, rinsed
- 1 tsp. sea salt
- 2 Tbsp. olive oil

Directions:
1. Preheat Air Fryer to 330 degrees F.
2. Line baking dish with parchment paper. Layer pork rind on baking sheet.
3. Drizzle in olive oil over pork rind. Season with salt. Put baking dish inside the Air Fryer basket. Cook for 30 minutes or until crisp.
4. Cool cracklings before slicing into bite-sized pieces. Serve

Recipe #57 - Soufflé

Ingredients:
- 4 egg yolks
- 5 egg whites
- 1 cup milk
- 1 oz. sugar
- 1 vanilla bean
- 1/4 cup softened butter
- ¼ cup all-purpose flour
- 1 teaspoon cream of tartar
- 2 teaspoons vanilla extract

Directions:
1. Preheat the Air Fryer to 330 degrees F.
2. Put together all-purpose flour and butter in a bowl. Mix well.
3. Meanwhile, pour milk in a saucepan. Add in sugar. Stir mixture well.
4. Put vanilla bean. Bring mixture to a boil. Add in the flour and butter mixture. Whisk until smooth.

5. Reduce the heat and allow to simmer until the mixture thickens.
6. Remove from heat. Discard vanilla bean. Place on an ice bath and let cool for 10 minutes.
7. Meanwhile, grease ramekins with butter. Sprinkle an equal amount of sugar. Beat egg yolks in a bowl. Add in milk mixture and vanilla extract. Mix well.
8. In another bowl, whisk cream of tartar, egg whites, and sugar until stiff peaks form. Fold in egg whites. Transfer the mixture into the prepared ramekins.
9. Place 2 ramekins inside the Air Fryer basket. Cook for 15 minutes.
10. **Sprinkle powdered sugar. Drizzle in chocolate sauce. Serve.**

Recipe #58 - Pumpkin and Maple Cupcakes
Ingredients:

- 2 tsp. pumpkin pie spice
- 1 cup of all-purpose flour, sifted

- 1/2 cup canned pumpkin puree
- 2 eggs
- 1 1/2 teaspoon vanilla extract
- 1/2 teaspoon baking powder
- Pinch of sea salt
- 1 stick butter, unsalted
- 1/2 cup sugar

For the frosting
- 2 tbsp. butter, unsalted
- 2 tsp. maple extract
- 2 cups powdered sugar, sifted
- 1 package cream cheese

Directions:
1. Preheat the Air Fryer to 350 degrees F.
2. Line 4 muffin cups with cupcake liner.
3. Sift the flour together with pumpkin pie spice, baking powder, and salt. Set aside.
4. Meanwhile, combine sugar and softened butter and sugar in another bowl. Add in eggs, vanilla extract, and pumpkin puree. Whisk well using a stand mixer until fluffy.
5. Tip in the flour with pumpkin pie spice mixture. Mix until well-combined.

6. Fill muffin cup with just the right amount of the batter. Place at least 4 muffin cups into the Air Fryer basket. Cook for 12 minutes.
7. Repeat the same cooking procedure with the rest of the cupcakes.
8. Place in a wire rack to let the cooked cupcakes cool.
9. While cooling, put together butter, cream cheese, maple extract, and powdered sugar in a small mixing bowl.
10. Top each cupcake with the maple cream cheese frosting. Serve.

Recipe #59 - Corn Rolls
Ingredients:

- 3 tablespoons of 3 colored capsicums, chopped finely
- 1 cup cream-style corn
- 1 onion, chopped finely
- 1 tablespoon olive oil

- 1 green chili, minced
- 1 teaspoon vinegar
- 1 teaspoon tomato ketchup
- Pinch of salt
- Pinch of pepper, to taste
- 4 bread slices, sides cut

- 1 teaspoon black sesame seeds, for garnish
- 1 tablespoon white sesame seeds, for garnish

Sealing paste
- 2 teaspoons maida (dissolved in 2 teaspoons of water)

Directions:
1. Preheat the Air Fryer to 320 degrees F.
2. Preheat a pan on a stove over medium-high flame. Add oil. Saute onions for 3 minutes. Stir in the green chili, capsicums, ketchup, pepper, salt, vinegar, and corn. Cook for 4 minutes while stirring often.
3. Transfer to a bowl and leave to cool.
4. Use a rolling pin to flatten the bread slices. Set aside.

5. Prepare the sealing paste. Put enough coating batter for the complete roll in a bowl. Add the corn mixture near the edge, roll it out, and make sure it's tight. Stick the ends using the sealing paste. Spray the rolls with a bit of water and coat them with sesame seeds. Wrap in a cling film and put in the fridge.
6. Cut each roll into 2 and place them in the cooking basket of the fryer. Cook for 10 minutes. Flip the rolls and cook for 10 more minutes.
7. Serve at once along with the sauce and lemon wedges.

Recipe #60 - Falafel with Cashew
Ingredients:
- ¾ cup canned chickpeas
- 3 Tbsp. almond flour
- 2 garlic cloves, chopped
- ¼ cup garlic roasted cashew nuts
- 1 shallot, peeled, minced

- 1 serving flax
- ¼ cup fresh cilantro, minced, reserve some for garnish
- Pinch of salt
- Pinch of white pepper, to taste

Directions:
1. Preheat Air Fryer to 330 degrees F.
2. Pour remaining ingredients into blender; process until chickpeas are mashed and batter comes together.
3. Roll into 8 large balls or 12 smaller ones; flatten these to make cooking go faster.
4. Place snap beans in the Air Fryer basket. Fry falafel in oil until crisp and golden brown on all sides. Drain on paper towels. Serve with fresh cilantro.

Bonus Recipe

Pork and Shrimp Siomai
Ingredients:

Seasoned soy sauce
- 2 Tbsp. light soy sauce
- ¼ tsp. roasted sesame oil
- ⅛ tsp. white sugar
- 1 Tbsp. lime juice, freshly squeezed

Filling
- ½ cup shrimps, chopped
- ⅛ cup carrots, diced
- ½ cup lean ground pork
- ⅛ cup jicama, diced
- ⅛ cup chives, chopped
- Pinch of sea salt, add more if needed
- Pinch of black pepper, to taste
- ⅛ tsp. rice wine

- 10 pieces square wonton wrappers, separated

Directions:
1. Preheat the Air Fryer to 300 degrees °F.
2. For the seasoned soy sauce, pour light soy sauce, sugar, sesame oil, and lime juice ingredients in a bowl. Stir well.

3. For the siomai, put together lean ground pork, carrots, shrimps, chives, salt, pepper and rice wine.
4. Place inside the food processor. Process mixture until a coarse paste is achieved.
5. Scoop just the right amount of filling on wonton wrappers. Press down on the filling and squeeze dumpling sides. Pinch and tap until the dumpling can stand on its own. Transfer to a baking sheet.
6. Repeat the same procedure until all fillings and wrappers are used up. Place inside the freezer for 2 hours.
7. Place dumplings into the Air Fryer basket. Cook for 10 minutes. Remove from the basket.
8. Serve with seasoned soy sauce on the side.

Sweet and Spicy Potato Sticks
Ingredients:
Spice mix
- Dash of nutmeg powder
- 1 tsp. cinnamon powder
- Dash of ginger powder
- ½ tsp. all spice powder

- Pinch of sea salt

- 2 sweet potatoes, sliced into inch thick matchsticks
- ⅛ cup honey

  Directions:

1. Preheat Air Fryer to 330 degrees F.
2. Line 2 baking sheets with aluminum foil. Combine spice mix ingredients in a small bowl. Place sweet potatoes flat but spaced apart on baking sheets. Drizzle in oil.
3. Put baking sheet in the Air fryer basket. Fry for 30 to 45 minutes. Remove from heat; place veggies into bowl with spice mix. Toss combine. Serve.

Conclusion

Thank you again for downloading this book!

I hope this book was able to help you know the many recipes that you can cook using the Air Fryer. This cooking appliance can also be a perfect alternative for your other cooking equipment. Think of it as an appliance that can do the role of frying, broiling, grilling, and even baking!

The next step is to try out the recipes here or make your own. The Air Fryer machine lets you cook your food in a healthy way with just few press of a button. This book contains delicious recipes that are quick to prepare and very easy to do.

Thank you once again for downloading this book. Good luck!

Part 2

Introduction

Preparing your favorite home meals is an integral part of everyday life. Barbecue wings, French fries, hamburgers – it's difficult to imagine modern life without these dishes. However, most of these dishes are harmful to our health because of the high content of fats and cholesterol. Constantly eating these dishes can cause heart problems, excessive weight and other difficulties. This is all due to the large amount of oil that is used when frying.

Solve this problem, reduce the amount of fat and at the same time get delicious food will allow a unique kitchen unit – the air fryer. This is a modern device, which is available in almost every kitchen, but many of us still do not know how to use it and what benefits it can bring to our life.

An air fryer is a kitchen appliance that cooks by circulating hot air around the food. A mechanical fan circulates the hot air around the food at high speed, cooking the food and producing a crispy layer via the Maillard effect.

Traditional frying methods induce the Maillard effect by completely submerging foods in hot oil. The air fryer works alternatively by coating the desired food in a thin layer of oil while circulating air heated up to 400-450 °F to confer energy and initiate the reaction. By doing this the appliance is able to fry foods like potato chips, chicken, fish, steak, French fries or pastries while using between 70% and 80% less oil than a traditional deep-fryer. This is great for your health and can significantly lower the level of cholesterol in the blood and reduce belly fat. In other words, air fryer is a must-have appliance in contemporary kitchen. So clean the dust from your air fryer and let's start creating! In this cookbook you'll find numerous air fryer recipes for you and your family to prepare amazing and easy air fryer recipes for any budget!

Cooking Measurement Conversion Chart

Liquid Measures

- 1 gal = 4 qt = 8 pt = 16 cups = 128 fl oz
- ½ gal = 2 qt = 4 pt = 8 cups = 64 fl oz
- ¼ gal = 1 qt = 2 pt = 4 cups = 32 fl oz
- ½ qt = 1 pt = 2 cups = 16 fl oz
- ¼ qt = ½ pt = 1 cup = 8 fl oz

Dry Measures

- 1 cup = 16 Tbsp = 48 tsp = 250ml
- ¾ cup = 12 Tbsp = 36 tsp = 175ml
- ⅔ cup = 10 ⅔ Tbsp = 32 tsp = 150ml
- ½ cup = 8 Tbsp = 24 tsp = 125ml
- ⅓ cup = 5 ⅓ Tbsp = 16 tsp = 75ml
- ¼ cup = 4 Tbsp = 12 tsp = 50ml
- ⅛ cup = 2 Tbsp = 6 tsp = 30ml
- 1 Tbsp = 3 tsp = 15ml

Dash or Pinch or Speck = less than ⅛ tsp

Quickies

- 1 fl oz = 30 ml
- 1 oz = 28.35 g
- 1 lb = 16 oz (454 g)
- 1 kg = 2.2 lb
- 1 quart = 2 pints

U.S.	Canadian
¼ tsp	1.25 mL
½ tsp	2.5 mL
1 tsp	5 mL
1 Tbl	15 mL
¼ cup	50 mL
⅓ cup	75 mL
½ cup	125 mL
⅔ cup	150 mL
¾ cup	175 mL
1 cup	250 mL
1 quart	1 liter

Recipe Abbreviations

- Cup = c or C
- Fluid = fl
- Gallon = gal
- Ounce = oz
- Package = pkg.
- Pint = pt
- Pound = lb or #
- Quart = qt
- Square = sq
- Tablespoon = T or Tbl or TBSP or TBS
- Teaspoon = t or tsp

Fahrenheit (°F) to Celsius (°C)

°F	°C
32 °F	0 °C
40 °F	4 °C
140 °F	60 °C
150 °F	65 °C
160 °F	70 °C
225 °F	107 °C
250 °F	121 °C
275 °F	135 °C
300 °F	150 °C
325 °F	165 °C
350 °F	177 °C
375 °F	190 °C
400 °F	205 °C
425 °F	220 °C
450 °F	230 °C
475 °F	245 °C
500 °F	260 °C

OVEN TEMPERATURES

- WARMING 200 °F
- VERY SLOW: 250 °F - 275 °F
- SLOW 300 °F - 325 °F
- MODERATE: 350 °F - 375 °F
- HOT 400 °F - 425 °F
- VERY HOT: 450 °F - 475 °F

Breakfast Recipes

Baked Eggs in Avocado Nests

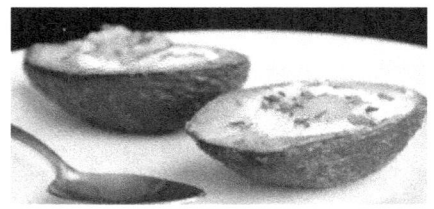

Prep time: 5 minutes
Cook time: 20 minutes
Servings: 2

Ingredients

- 1 large avocado, halved
- 2 eggs
- 4 grape tomato, halved
- 2 teaspoon chives, chopped
- A pinch of sea salt and black pepper

Directions

1. Cut avocado in half length-wise. Remove the pit and widen the hole in

each half by scraping out the avocado flesh with the help of the spoon.
2. Place avocado halves in a small oven proof baking dish cut side up.
3. Beat an egg into each half of avocado. Season with salt and pepper.
4. Cook for about 10-15 minutes in 370°F into the Air Fryer.
5. Top with grape tomato halves and chives. Enjoy!

Fried Eggs with Ham

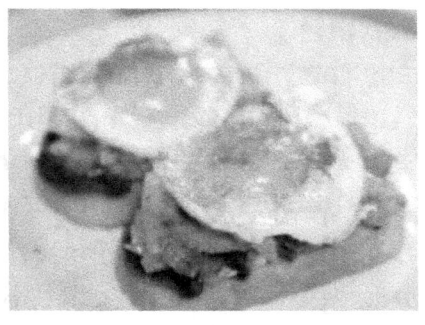

Prep time: 5 minutes
Cook time: 10-15 minutes
Servings: 4
Ingredients
- 4 large eggs
- 2 oz (nearly 2 thin slices) ham
- 2 teaspoon butter
- 2 tablespoon heavy cream
- 3 tablespoon parmesan cheese, grated
- 2 teaspoon fresh chives, chopped
- A pinch of smoked paprika
- Salt and ground black pepper to taste

Directions
1. Grease the pie pan with butter and line the bottom with ham slices. Make the bottom and sides of the pie pan completely covered with ham.
2. In a small bowl beat 1 egg, add heavy cream, a pinch of salt and 1/8 teaspoon ground pepper. Whisk to combine.

3. Pour this egg mixture over the ham and beat remaining 3 eggs over top.
4. Season with salt and ground pepper, sprinkle with parmesan cheese.
5. Preheat the Air Fryer to 320-350 F
6. Place the pie pan into the cooking basket and cook for 12 minutes.
7. When finished, remove fried eggs from the pie pan with the help of spatula and transfer to the plate. Season with smoked paprika and chopped chives

Air Fryer Spinach Frittata

Prep time: 5 minutes
Cook time: 10-12 minutes
Servings: 2
Ingredients
- 1 small onion, minced
- 1/3 pack (4oz) spinach
- 3 eggs, beaten
- 3 oz mozzarella cheese
- 1 tablespoon olive oil
- Salt and pepper to taste

Directions
1. Preheat the Air fryer to 370 F

2. In a baking pan heat the oil for about a minute.
3. Add minced onions into the pan and cook for 2-3 minutes.
4. Add spinach and cook for about 3-5 minutes to about half cooked. They may look a bit dry but it is ok, just keep frying with the oil.
5. In the large bowl whisk the beaten eggs, season with salt and pepper and sprinkle with cheese. Pour the mixture into a baking pan.
6. Place the pan in the air fryer and cook for 6-8 minutes or until cooked.

Easy Breakfast Casserole

Prep time: 15 minutes
Cook time: 25-30 minutes
Servings: 5-6

Ingredients

- 1 pound hot breakfast sausage
- ½ bag (15 oz) frozen hash browns, shredded
- 1 cups cheddar cheese, shredded
- 4 eggs
- 1 cup milk
- ¼ teaspoon pepper
- ¼ teaspoon garlic powder
- ¼ teaspoon onion powder
- ½ teaspoon salt

Directions

1. In the large skillet cook sausages until no longer pink. Drain fat.
2. Add shredded hash browns to the skillet and cook until lightly brown.
3. Place hash browns in the bottom of oven proof pan, lightly greased. Top with sausages and cheese.

4. It the bowl whisk together eggs, salt, pepper, garlic powder, onion powder, and milk.
5. Pour egg mixture over the hash browns.
6. Preheat the Air Fryer to 350-370 F
7. Place the pan in the fryer into the fryer and cook for 25-30 minutes, until become ready.

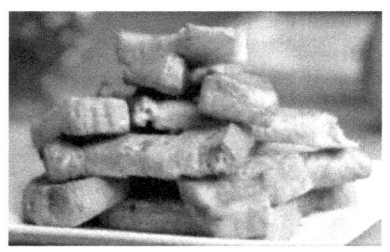

French Toast Sticks

Prep time: 5 minutes
Cook time: 5-8 minutes
Servings: 2

Ingredients
- 4 pieces bread, sliced
- 2 tablespoon soft butter

- 2 eggs, beaten
- ¼ teaspoon cinnamon
- ¼ teaspoon nutmeg
- ¼ teaspoon ground cloves
- Icing sugar for garnish
- A pinch of salt

Directions

1. It the bowl beat two eggs, sprinkle with salt, cinnamon, nutmeg and ground cloves.
2. Butter both sides of bread and cut into stripes.
3. Preheat the Air Fryer to 350-370 F
4. Dip each bread strip into the egg mixture and then put into the air fryer.
5. Cook for about 5-8 minutes until eggs are cooked and bread become golden.
6. Garnish with icing sugar and top with cream or maple syrup (as for your desire).

Side & Entrees

Green Beans with Shallots and Almonds

Prep time: 5 minutes
Cook time: 25 minutes
Servings: 4-5

Ingredients

- 1½ pound French green beans, stems removed
- ½ pound shallots, peeled, stems removed and cut into quarters
- ¼ cup slivered almonds, lightly roasted
- 2 tablespoon olive oil
- 1 tablespoon salt
- ½ teaspoon black pepper, ground

Directions

1. Bring water to a boil over high heat. Once boiling, add the green beans, season with salt and cook for 2 minutes. Remove from the water and drain in a colander.
2. Mix cooked beans with quartered shallots, some additional salt and

black pepper and sprinkle with the olive oil. Toss well to coat evenly.
3. Cook bean mixture for 25 minutes at 390 F tossing them twice throughout the cooking process. The green beans should be lightly browned and tender once cooked.
4. Transfer cooked beans to a serving platter.

Fried Carrots with Cumin

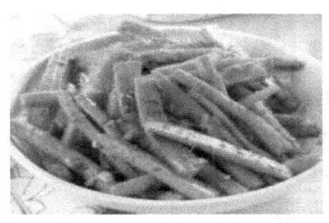

Prep time: 5 minutes
Cook time: 20 minutes
Servings: 4
Ingredients
- 1 pound carrots, peeled

- 1 tablespoon olive oil
- 1 teaspoon cumin seeds
- 1 handful of fresh coriander, crushed
- A pinch of salt

Directions
1. Wash the carrots.
2. Drizzle carrots with olive oil. Sprinkle with cumin seeds and stir to combine.
3. Cook the carrots in the air fryer for approximately 20 minutes at 360 F, until lightly browned and tender.
4. Scatter with crushed coriander.

Cheesy French Fries

Prep time: 7 minutes
Cook time: 25 minutes
Servings: 4
Ingredients
- 2 pounds potatoes, cut into strips
- 1/2 teaspoon dried thyme
- A pinch rosemary dried and crumbled
- 1 tablespoon olive oil

- 1/2 cup grated parmesan

Directions
1. Cut potatoes into nearly ¼ inch x 3-inch stripes and dry them using a paper towel.
2. Preheat your air fryer to 330-350°F.
3. Sprinkle potatoes with olive oil, thyme, and rosemary.
4. Cook in the air fryer for 20-25 minutes, until golden and crispy.
5. Serve and top with grated parmesan.

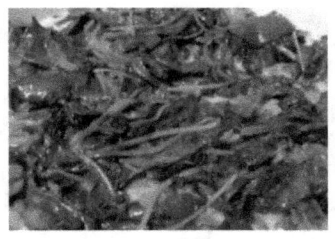

Spinach with Bacon, Onion & Garlic
Prep time: 5 minutes
Cook time: 10 minutes
Servings: 4
Ingredients
- 6 oz spinach
- 2 bacon strips
- 1 small onion, cut

- 1 garlic clove, minced

Directions
1. Cut onion and bacon, mince garlic.
2. Preheat the air fryer to 350 F.
3. Cook onion and bacon for 2-3 minutes.
4. Add spinach and cook another 5-7 minutes, until ready and tender.

Feta Pillows
Prep time: 10 minutes
Cook time: 20 minutes
Servings: 4-5
Ingredients
- 1 egg yolk
- 2 tablespoons chopped parsley
- 4 ounces feta cheese
- 1 finely chopped scallion
- 2 finely chopped sheets of frozen pastry
- 2 tablespoons olive oil
- Ground black pepper to taste

Directions

1. Mix beat egg yolk with feta, scallion, parsley and pepper in a bowl.
2. Each sheet of filo cut into three strips.
3. This pasta put with a spoon in the strip of pastry and make a pillow or triangle.
4. Cook in air fryer at 390 F for 3 minutes and then cook on 360 F for 2 minutes.

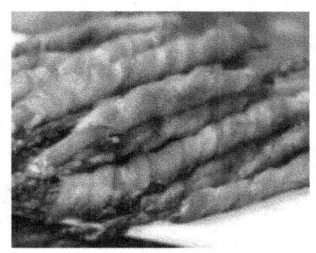

Asparagus Spears Rolled with Bacon
Prep time: 10 minutes
Cook time: 9 minutes
Servings: 3-4
Ingredients
- 1 bundle asparagus, 20-25 spears
- 4 slices bacon
- 1 garlic clove, crushed
- 1 tablespoon olive oil
- 1 ½ tablespoon brown sugar

- ½ tablespoon toasted sesame seeds

Directions
1. Combine olive oil, brown sugar, and crushed garlic.
2. Separate bundle of asparagus into four equal-sized bunches and wrap each in a bacon slice.
3. Cover asparagus bunches with oil mixture.
4. Preheat the Air Fryer to 340-360 F
5. Put bunches into the air fryer and sprinkle with sesame seeds.
6. Cook for approximately 8 minutes.

Rice and Vegetable Stuffed Tomatoes
Prep time: 12 minutes
Cook time 25 minutes
Servings: 3
Ingredients
- 3 tomatoes, cored
- 2 cups white rice, cooked
- 1 medium onion, diced
- 1 medium carrot, diced
- 1 tablespoon olive oil
- 2 garlic cloves, minced
- Ground pepper

- Salt

Directions

1. Sprinkle the olive oil in a skillet and sauté carrot, onion, and garlic for 2-3 minutes; season the mixture with salt and pepper.
2. Add cooked rice to the vegetable mixture, stir to combine.
3. Preheat the Air Fryer to 340 F.
4. Fill in cored tomatoes with mixture.
5. Place stuffed tomatoes into the air fryer and cook for 20-25 minutes.

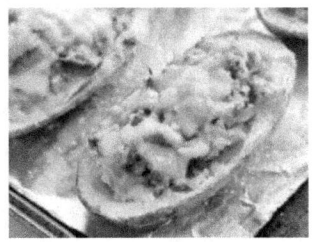

Potato Halves with Bacon and Herbs
Prep time: 5 minutes
Cook time: 25-35 minutes
Servings: 4
Ingredients
- 4 middle-sized potatoes, peeled and halved

- 6 garlic cloves, minced
- 4 slices bacon, cut into 1-inch pieces
- 2 sprigs rosemary, crushed
- 1 tablespoon olive oil
- ¼ teaspoon black pepper, freshly ground
- A pinch of salt

Instructions
1. Preheat your Air fryer to 370 F.
2. Combine halved potatoes, minced garlic, rosemary, and bacon pieces. Sprinkle the mixture with olive oil, season with salt and pepper. Mix well.
3. Put everything in the air fryer basket and cook for 25-30 minutes, or until golden brown.

Cheese & Bacon Muffins
Prep time: 8 minutes
Cook time: 30 minutes
Servings: 4-6
Ingredients
- 1 - ½ cup all-purpose flour

- 1 large egg, beaten
- 3-4 large bacon slices
- 1 medium-sized onion, sliced
- ½ cup cheese, shredded
- 2 teaspoon baking powder
- 2 tablespoon vegetable oil
- 1 cup skimmed milk
- 1 teaspoon parsley, dried and crushed
- 1/8 teaspoon black pepper, ground
- A pinch of salt to taste

Directions

1. Preheat the sauté pan over the medium-high heat and cook the bacon. When it's almost done add the onion and cook for couple minutes, until transparent and set aside.
2. Combine parsley, baking powder, all-purpose flour, and grated cheese. Then add milk, vegetable oil, egg and cooked bacon with onion. Mix with the wooden spoon until it becomes a sticky to thick dough.
3. Drain the oil from your bacon and onion and also add to the mixture.

4. Preheat the Air Fryer to 390 F. Spoon the mixture into six medium sized muffin cases and cook in the Air Fryer for 20 minutes. Then, reduce the temperature to 350 F and cook additionally for 8-10 minutes to make sure they are cooked in the center. Work in batches to finish all muffins.

Asparagus Spears Rolled with Bacon

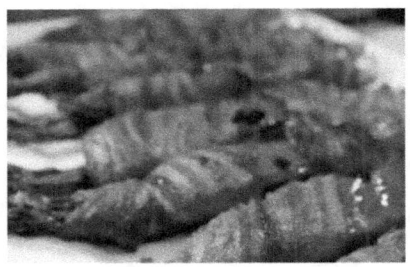

Prep time: 10 minutes
Cook time: 9 minutes
Servings: 3-4

Ingredients

- 1 bundle asparagus, 20-25 spears
- 4 slices bacon
- 1 garlic clove, crushed
- 1 tablespoon olive oil
- 1 ½ tablespoon brown sugar
- ½ tablespoon toasted sesame seeds

Directions

1. Combine olive oil, brown sugar, and crushed garlic.
2. Separate bundle of asparagus into four equal-sized bunches and wrap each in a bacon slice.
3. Cover asparagus bunches with oil mixture.
4. Preheat the Air Fryer to 340-360 F
5. Put bunches into the air fryer and sprinkle with sesame seeds.
6. Cook for approximately 8 minutes.

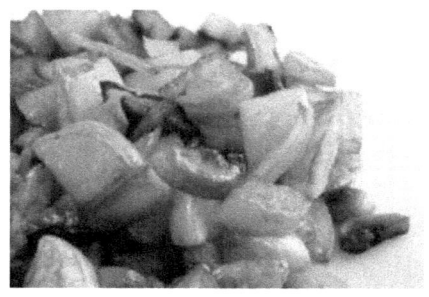

Fried Potatoes with Mushrooms
Prep time: 5 minutes
Cook time: 25 minutes
Servings: 4

Ingredients
- 1 - ½ pound potatoes, peeled
- 5 oz mushrooms
- 1 medium onion, chopped
- 1 tablespoon spoon olive oil
- Salt to taste

Directions
1. Peel potatoes and cut them into 1-inch cubes.
2. Cut mushrooms into quarters.
3. Preheat the air fryer to 350 F, sprinkle cooking basket with olive oil and cook onion for 2-3 minutes.
4. Add potato cubes, season with salt to taste and cook for 10-15 minutes, until potato cubes are nearly cooked.
5. Add mushroom quarters to the air fryer and cook for 2 minutes.

Potato Chips

Prep time: 5 minutes
Cook time: 22 minutes
Servings: 2

Ingredients

- 2 large russet potatoes
- ½ tablespoon extra virgin olive oil
- Salt to taste

Directions

1. Peel and slice the potatoes thinly.
2. Soak slices in a bowl of cold water for 30 minutes; change the water halfway through and give the slices a good mix.
3. Cook potato slices for about 20 minutes at 390 F.
4. When ready, replace chips in the large plate, season with salt to taste and serve.

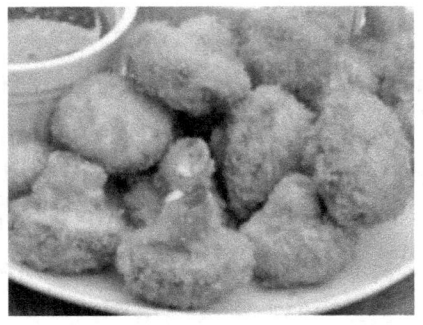

Breaded Mushrooms

Prep time: 10 minutes
Cook time: 10 minutes
Servings: 2-3

Ingredients

- 10 oz button mushrooms
- ¼ cup flour
- 1 egg
- ½ cup breadcrumbs
- 3 oz cheese, finely grated
- Salt and pepper for seasoning

Directions

1. Mix breadcrumbs with cheese, season with salt and pepper to taste and set aside.

2. In another middle bowl beat an egg and also set aside.
3. Preheat the Air Fryer to 340-360 F
4. Roll mushrooms in the flour, dip them into the beaten egg and dip in the breadcrumbs and cheese mixture.
5. Cook in the air fryer for 7-10 minutes. Shake once while cooking.

Brussels Sprout with Bacon

Prep time: 5 minutes
Cook time: 15 minutes
Servings: 3

Ingredients

- 1 strip bacon, diced
- 1 pound Brussels sprouts
- ¼ cup water
- 1 tablespoon freshly squeezed lemon juice
- ½ tablespoon extra virgin olive oil
- Salt and freshly ground pepper to taste

Directions

1. Preheat air fryer to 340-360°F.

2. Cook diced bacon for 7 minutes.
3. Trim the bottom of each Brussels sprout, pull off outer leaves and slice the core into quarters.
4. Add Brussels sprout leaves and quarters into the air fryer and drizzle with water. Cook for nearly 7 minutes.
5. Serve, sprinkle with fresh lemon juice and olive oil, and season to taste with salt and pepper.

Poultry Recipes

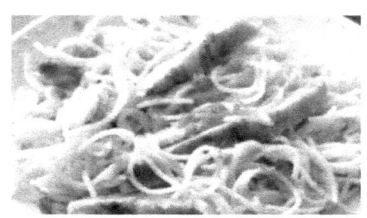

Chicken with Spaghetti

Prep time: 5 minutes
Cook time: 15 minutes
Servings: 3

Ingredients

- 1 pound chicken tenders
- ¾ cup soy sauce
- ½ cup mirin
- 1 tablespoon grated ginger
- 1 medium carrot, chopped
- 2 small onions, sliced
- 1 pack spaghetti
- Salt and pepper to taste

Directions

1. Cut chicken into bite-size pieces and place in the round baking tray.
2. Add sugar, soy sauce, mirin, grated ginger, carrots, and onions. Mix well.
3. Place the baking tray to the air fryer and cook for about 15 minutes at 320 F.
4. Meanwhile, cook spaghetti in salted water.
5. When ready, mix chicken with spaghetti and serve.

Crispy Fried Wings

Prep time: 10 minutes
Cook time: 15 minutes
Servings: 6

Ingredients

- 3 pounds chicken wings
- 2 tablespoons soy sauce
- 2 tablespoons olive oil
- 6 garlic cloves, finely chopped
- 1 finely chopped habanera pepper, without seeds and ribs
- 1 teaspoon cinnamon

- 1 teaspoon white pepper
- 1 tablespoon all spice
- 1 teaspoon cayenne pepper
- 1 teaspoon salt
- 1 tablespoon finely chopped fresh thyme
- 2 tablespoons brown sugar
- 4 finely chopped scallions
- 1 tablespoons grated fresh ginger
- 5 tablespoons lime juice
- ½ cup red wine vinegar

Directions

1. All ingredients mix in a large mixing bowl. Dip chicken wings in the marinade and set aside for at least 2 hours.
2. Preheat the air fryer to 390 F.
3. Cook wings in the air fryer for 16-18 minutes. Shake couple of times during the cooking.

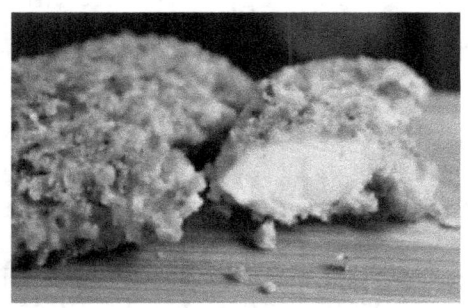

Breaded Chicken Tenders

Prep time: 10 minutes
Cook time: 15 minutes
Servings: 3

Ingredients

- 1 pound chicken tenders
- 2 beaten eggs
- ½ teaspoon salt
- ½ breadcrumbs
- ½ cup flour
- 2 tablespoons olive oil
- 1 teaspoon black pepper

Directions

1. Preheat the air fryer to 340 F.
2. Prepare three bowls – first one with breadcrumbs combined with oil, the

second one for eggs and the third for flour.
3. Roll the chicken in flour, then in eggs and finally into breadcrumbs.
4. Cook in the fryer for 10 minutes on 330 F, then turn up the temperature to 390 F and cook another 5 minutes. The chicken should have golden brown.

Chicken Breasts with Cream Sauce

Prep time: 5-7 minutes
Cook time: 15-18 minutes
Servings: 2-3

Ingredients
- 2 chicken breasts, skinless and boneless
- ½ cup cream
- ½ tablespoon olive oil
- A pinch salt and ground pepper

Directions
1. Combine cream, olive oil, season with salt and ground pepper.

2. Preheat the Air Fryer to 350°F.
3. Dip the chicken breasts into the cream mixture. Make sure that all sides are in the mixture.
4. Replace meat in the fryer and cook for 15 minutes or until golden and ready.

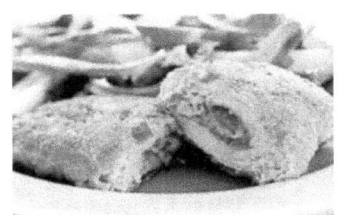

Sausage Stuffed in Chicken Fillet
Prep time: 5 minutes
Cook time: 15 minutes
Servings: 4
Ingredients
- 4 sausages you prefer
- 4 chicken fillets (thigh or breast)
- 8 bamboo skewers or toothpicks

Directions

1. Push and roll chicken meat with a rolling pin.
2. Remove sausage casing.
3. Place sausage meat into the chicken filet.
4. Fold chicken meat into halves and seal by 2 toothpicks into each piece.
5. Preheat the Air Fryer to 390 F, place meat into the frying basket and cook for 15 minutes.
6. Serve with any dipping sauce you like.

Crispy Chicken Fillet with Cheese
Prep time: 10 minutes
Cook time: 15 minutes
Servings: 4-5
Ingredients
- 2 pounds chicken tenders
- ½ cup parmesan cheese
- 1 cup breadcrumbs
- 1 oz butter, melted
- 1 egg
- 1 teaspoon garlic powder

- 1 teaspoon Italian herbs

Directions

1. Mix beaten egg, melted butter, garlic powder and, Italian herbs.
2. Marinate chicken tenders into the mixture for at least 30 minutes.
3. I another bowl mix breadcrumbs with parmesan cheese.
4. Cover chicken meat with breadcrumb mixture.
5. Cook chicken in the air fryer for 5-6 minutes at 350 F. Then flip to another side and cook for another 3-5 minutes, until chicken becomes golden and ready.

Korean Chicken

Prep time: 10 minutes
Cook time: 13 minutes
Servings: 3
Ingredients

- 1 pound chicken breasts
- 3 garlic cloves, crushed
- 1 tablespoon grated ginger
- ¼ teaspoon ground black pepper
- ½ cup soy sauce

- ½ cup pineapple juice
- 1 tablespoon olive oil
- 2 tablespoon sesame seeds

Directions
1. Mix all ingredients in the large bowl.
2. Cut chicken breasts and soak in the marinade. Set aside for at least 30-40 minutes.
3. Cook marinated chicken in the air fryer at 380 F for about 10-15 minutes.
4. Sprinkle cooked chicken with sesame seeds and serve.

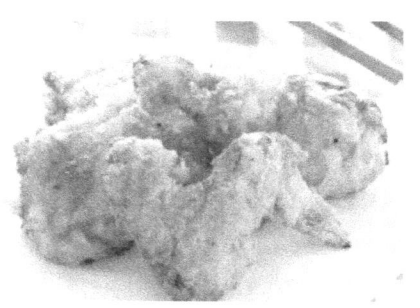

Classic Crispy Chicken Wings
Prep time: 5 minutes
Cook time: 35 minutes
Servings: 4-5

Ingredients
- 1 pound chicken wings
- 2 tablespoon Provencal herbs
- 1 teaspoon black ground pepper
- Salt to taste

Directions
1. Evenly coat chicken wings with salt, ground pepper, and Provencal herbs. Mix with hands.
2. Preheat the Air Fryer to 370-390 F
3. Spray the cooking basket with a nonstick coating.
4. Place coated wings into the air fryer basket and cook for 15-20 minutes. Shake couple times during cooking.
5. Serve with your favorite dipping sauce (I prefer BBQ but Buffalo, Ranch or Blue Cheese is also OK). Enjoy!

Chicken Tenders with Honey
Prep time: 20 minutes
Cook time: 10-12 minutes

Servings: 3

Ingredients

- 1 pound chicken tenders, skinless and boneless
- ¼ cup water
- 1/2 teaspoon red pepper flakes
- 3 tablespoon tamari (aged soy sauce)
- 2 tablespoon honey
- 2 gloves of garlic, minced
- 1 tablespoon ginger, peeled and grated
- ¾ cup green onions, thinly sliced

Directions

1. Mix water, white parts of onion, soy sauce, honey, garlic and ginger.
2. Cut chicken tenders into stripe pieces and toss into marinade at least for 30 minutes or more.
3. Pour entire mixture into the air fryer and cook at 350 F for about 5-10 minutes.
4. Sprinkle with green parts of onion as decoration and serve.

Delicious Meat Recipes

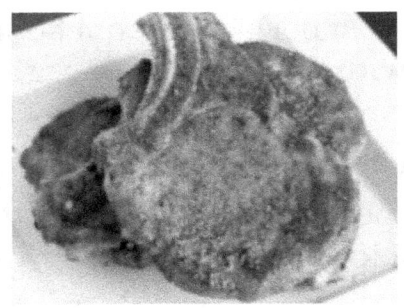

Pork Chop

Prep time: 15 minutes
Cook time: 15 minutes
Servings: 2

Ingredients

- 2 middle pieces pork chop
- 1 tablespoon plain flour
- 1 egg, beaten
- 2 tablespoon olive oil
- 3 tablespoon breadcrumbs
- Salt and ground pepper for seasoning

Directions
1. Season pork chops with salt and ground pepper from both sides.
2. In three different bowls place plain flour, beaten egg, and breadcrumbs.
3. Coat each pork chop from both sides first with flour then with egg and with breadcrumbs.
4. Preheat the Air Fryer to 380 F
5. Cook pork chops for 10 minutes from one side and 5 minutes from another side.
6. Serve with cooked rice and mashed potatoes.

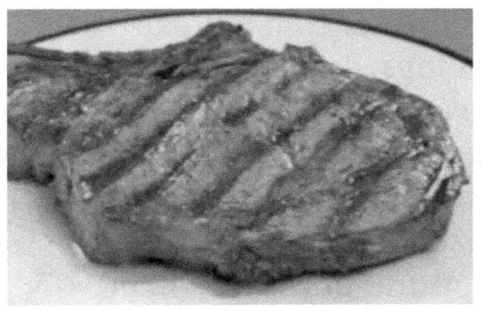

Rib Eye Steak

Prep time: 5 minutes
Cook time: 15-20 minutes
Servings: 4

Ingredients

- 2-pound rib eye steak
- 1 tablespoon steak rub
- 1 tablespoon olive oil

Directions

1. Preheat your Air Fryer to 390-400 F.
2. Season the steak on both sides with rub and sprinkle with olive oil.
3. Cook the steak for about 7-8 minutes, rotate the steak and cook for another 6-7 minute until golden brown and ready.

Fried Beef with Potatoes and Mushrooms
 Prep time: 20 minutes
 Cook time: 15 minutes
 Servings: 4-5
 Ingredients
- **1 pound beef steak**
- **1 medium onion, sliced**
- **8 oz mushrooms, sliced**
- **½ pound potatoes, diced**
- **Sauce you prefer (Barbecue or Teriyaki)**
- Salt and black pepper for seasoning

 Directions
1. **Chop onion and mushrooms, dice potatoes. Sprinkle them with salt and pepper.**
2. **Cut beef steak into 1 inch pieces.**
3. **Combine onion, potatoes, mushrooms and beef. Marinate with sauce and set aside for 15-20 minutes.**
4. **Preheat the Air Fryer to 350-370 F**
5. **Put meat and vegetables into the air fryer and cook for 15 minutes.**
6. After cooking replace the meal to the serving plate and sprinkle with fresh chopped parsley.

Pork Tenderloin

Prep time: 15 minutes
Cook time: 15 minutes
Servings: 2-3
Ingredients

- 1 pound pork tenderloin
- 1 medium red or yellow pepper, sliced
- 1 large red onion, sliced
- 2 tablespoon Provencal herbs
- 2 tablespoons olive oil
- ½ tablespoon mustard
- Ground black pepper
- Salt

Directions

1. Combine sliced pepper and onion, Provencal herbs, and olive oil; season with salt and ground pepper to taste.
2. Cut the pork tenderloin into 4-6 large pieces, scrub with salt, ground pepper, and mustard.
3. Preheat your air fryer to 370-390 F.

4. **Place vegetable mixture to the air fryer.**
5. **Coat meat pieces with olive oil and place them up to the vegetables.**
6. **Cook for 15 minutes until meat and vegetables will become roasted.**
7. Turn the meat and vegetable in the middle of cooking process.

Meatballs Stewed in Yogurt

Prep time: 10 minutes
Cook time: 20-25 minutes
Servings: 4
Ingredients

- **1 pound ground beef**
- **4 ounces ground turkey**
- **2 tablespoon parsley, finely chopped**
- **1 tablespoon mint, finely chopped**
- **1 teaspoon ground coriander**
- **1 teaspoon ground cumin**
- **1 teaspoon cayenne pepper**
- **2 garlic cloves, finely chopped**
- **2 tablespoon olive oil**
- **1 teaspoon red chili paste**
- **1 egg white**
- 1 teaspoon salt

Yogurt

- **½ cup non-fat yogurt**
- **2 tablespoons buttermilk**
- **¼ cup sour cream**
- 2 pinches salt

Directions

1. All ingredients for meatballs mix in a large bowl and roll the meatballs with hands. It should be the size of golf ball.
2. Cook them in Air fryer at 390 F for 6-8 minutes.
3. Meanwhile, combine all ingredients for yogurt in a bowl and mix them well. Serve meatballs with yogurt topping.

Cheese Stuffed Burgers

Prep time: 10 minutes
Cook time: 20 minutes
Servings: 3-4
Ingredients
- **1 pound finely ground beef**
- **2 oz cheddar cheese**
- Salt and ground pepper to taste

Directions
1. Break up minced beef and season with salt and black pepper.
2. Divide the mince into 4 balls.
3. Cut the cheese into 4 equal pieces.

4. **Take half mince from one of the balls and form it into a circle about 2.5-inch wide.**
5. **Push a piece of the cheese into the center of the mince ball.**
6. **From the remaining half of mince make the circle with the same width and put on the top. Carefully join the base with cheese and the top and then gently form the burger with your hands.**
7. **Preheat the Air Fryer to 370 F**
8. Cook burgers in the air fryer for about 15-20 minutes until they become ready turning halfway through the cooking time.

Fish & Seafood Recipes

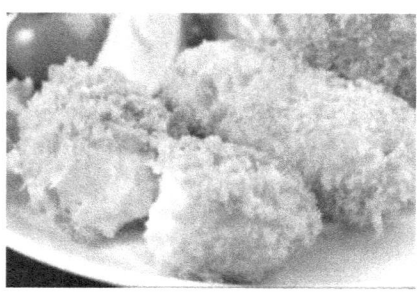

Crab Pillows

Prep time: 15 minutes
Cook time: 20 minutes
Servings: 4-5

Ingredients

- 2 egg whites
- 1 pound crab meat
- 2 tablespoons celery, finely chopped
- ¼ teaspoon tarragon, finely chopped
- ½ teaspoon parsley, finely chopped
- ¼ teaspoon chives, finely chopped
- 1 tablespoon olive oil
- 1 small red onion
- ½ teaspoon cayenne pepper

- ¼ cup sour cream
- ¼ cup mayonnaise

Breading

- 3 beaten eggs
- 1 cup breadcrumbs
- 1 cup flour
- ½ teaspoon salt

Directions

1. Mix onions, celery, peppers and olive oil in a small pan heated on medium-high. Cook for a couple of minutes, until the onion is translucent.
2. Combine breadcrumbs with olive oil and salt to a fine paste.
3. In three bowls prepare eggs, breadcrumbs, and flour. In special bowl mix mayonnaise, crab meat, sour cream, and egg whites.
4. Mold crab meat into balls, roll in flour, eggs and breadcrumbs and put in the air fryer, heated to 390°F, and cook 8-10 minutes.

Spring Rolls Stuffed with Shrimps

Prep time: 10 minutes
Cook time: 15 minutes
Servings: 4

Ingredients

- 4 oz shrimps, cooked
- 12 spring roll wrappers
- 1 teaspoon root ginger, freshly grated
- 2 oz mushrooms, sliced
- 1 egg, beaten
- 1 teaspoon Chinese five-spice powder
- 1 oz bean sprouts
- 1 spring onion
- 1 small carrot, cut into matchsticks
- 1 tablespoon groundnut oil
- 1 tablespoon soy sauce

Directions

1. In the large skillet or wok heat the oil over medium-high heat. Add ginger and mushrooms and cook for 2 minutes. Add the soy sauce, Chinese five-spice powder, bean sprouts, spring onions and carrots. Cook for 1 minute and then set

aside to chill. Add the shrimps and toss.
2. **Preheat the Air fryer to 370-390 F. Roll up the shrimp mixture in spring roll wrappers, sealing with beaten egg. Brush each roll with oil.**
3. Cook in batches in the air fryer basket for 5 minutes.

Yummy Shrimps with Bacon

Prep time: 10 minutes
Cook time: 15 minutes
Servings: 4
Ingredients
- **16 tiger shrimp, deveined**
- 1 pound (also 16 slices) thinly sliced bacon

Directions
1. Every shrimp wrap in bacon. Put shrimps in refrigerator for 20 minutes
2. Cook in Air fryer at 390°F for 5-7 minutes. Then just dry shrimps on paper towel.
3. Serve and enjoy.

Fried Crab Chips

Prep time: 7 minutes
Cook time: 12-13 minutes
Servings: 3-4
Ingredients
- **1 pack crabsticks (nearly 1 pound)**

- **2 tablespoon extra virgin olive oil**
- **2 teaspoon seasoning for you taste - I use curry or Italian seasoning**
- 1/3 cup Parmesan cheese, shredded (optional)

Directions
1. **First of all, preheat your Air Fryer to 380 F.**
2. **Cut the crab sticks lengthwise and shred into smaller, but not too small. 1 inch width would be good enough.**
3. **Sprinkle the Air Fryer basket with the olive oil, place crushed crab sticks and fry for 10-12 minutes until golden. Work in batches if you have many pieces.**
4. When ready, replace fried sticks in the plate, season slightly and sprinkle with shredded cheese.

Cod with Tomatoes

Prep time: 5 minutes
Cook time: 15 minutes
Servings: 4

Ingredients

- **4 cod fillets**
- **10-12 cherry tomatoes**
- **1 tablespoon olive oil**
- **Salt and pepper to taste**
- Basil, parsley or any other fresh herbs of your choice for garnish

Directions

1. **Season cod fillets with salt and pepper, sprinkle with olive oil and cook for 12 minutes in the air fryer at 360 F.**
2. **When almost done, add cherry tomatoes cut on halves. Cook for another 3-4 minutes.**
3. Serve cod fillets with grilled tomatoes and herbs of your choice.

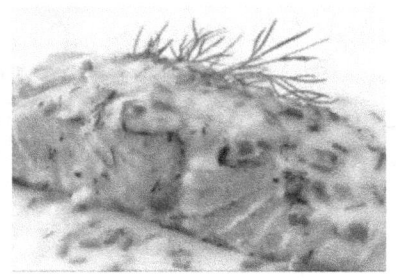

Salmon in Delicious Sauce

Prep time: 10 minutes
Cook time: 15 minutes
Servings: 4

Ingredients

- 1 pound salmon, cut (each should be 6 oz. and prepare 4 pieces)
- 2 teaspoons olive oil
- Salt to taste

Sauce

- ½ cup non-fat yogurt
- ½ cup sour cream
- 2 tablespoons finely chopped dill
- Salt to taste

Directions

1. Cut salmon into 4 equal pieces. Sprinkle each piece with oil and season with salt.

2. **Cook the salmon in the air fryer at 270°F for 15 minutes.**
3. Meanwhile, mix sour cream, yogurt, chopped dill and salt in large bowl and pour cooked salmon with this sauce.

Tender Tuna Nuggets

Prep time: 10 minutes
Cook time: 10 minutes
Servings: 4-5

Ingredients

- 2 cans tuna (10-12 oz)
- ½ cup breadcrumbs
- 3 tablespoon olive oil
- 2 tablespoon parsley, chopped
- 1 egg
- 2 teaspoon Dijon mustard
- Ground pepper
- Salt

Directions

1. Mix tuna, olive oil, parsley, egg and mustard in a large bowl.
2. Form tuna mixture into nuggets and place them on the baking sheet.
3. Cool nuggets in the fridge for 2 hours
4. Preheat the Air Fryer to 350 F.
5. Put frozen nuggets to the air fryer and cook for 10 minutes.

Cod Pillows

Prep time: 10 minutes
Cook time: 15 minutes
Servings: 4

Ingredients

- 1 pound cod
- 2 eggs, beaten
- 2 tablespoons olive oil
- 1 cup flour
- ¾ cup breadcrumbs
- A pinch of salt

Directions

1. Preheat the air fryer to 390°F.
2. Cut the cod into small parts, 1 inch in width and 2.5 inches in length.
3. Combine breadcrumbs with olive oil and season with salt.
4. In three bowls put eggs, a breadcrumbs mixture, and flour.
5. Roll cod into breadcrumbs, then in eggs and finally in flour. Put in the fryer.

6. Cook 8-10 minutes or until cod has a brown color.

Miso Tilapia

Prep time: 8 minutes
Cook time: 12 minutes
Servings: 4

Ingredients

- 1 pound tilapia fillet
- 2 garlic cloves, minced
- 1 scallion, sliced
- ½ cup miso
- ½ cup mirin
- 1 teaspoon grated ginger

Directions

1. Cut tilapia fillet into 4 equal pieces.
2. Combine miso, mirin, grated ginger, and crushed garlic in the bowl.
3. Soak fish fillets into this mixture and set aside for 20-30 minutes.
4. Cook tilapia in the air fryer for 10-12 minutes at 340 F.

5. Serve with sliced scallions.

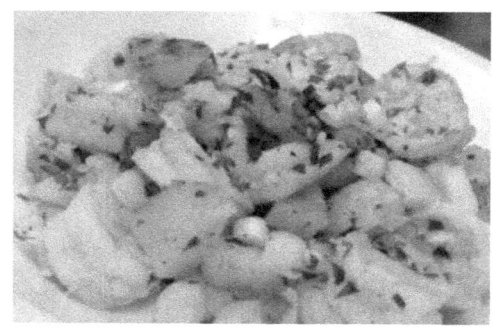

Potatoes with Garlic, Tomatoes and Shrimps

Prep time: 8 minutes
Cook time: 35 minutes
Servings: 4

Ingredients
- 1 - ½ pound small new potatoes, unpeeled
- 4 middle tomatoes
- 12 large shrimp, peeled
- 2 tablespoons chopped parsley
- 5 garlic cloves
- 2 tablespoons olive oil

- Salt and freshly ground pepper for seasoning

Directions
1. Wash and dry potatoes.
2. Separate garlic cloves without removing the peel.
3. Put potatoes and garlic in the air fryer and cook for 15 minutes at 340 F.
4. Add unpeeled tomatoes to the air fryer and cook for another 10 minutes.
5. Add the shrimps and herbs. Cook for 5 minutes or until shrimps will be ready.

Dessert Recipes

Indian Banana Chips

Prep time: 10 minutes
Cook time: 15 minutes
Servings: 2-3

Ingredients

- 4 raw bananas
- ½ teaspoon turmeric powder
- ½ teaspoon Chat Masala
- 1 teaspoon salt
- ½ cup water
- 1 teaspoon olive oil

Directions

1. Preheat your Air Fryer to 350 F
2. Combine turmeric powder and salt with water smoothly.
3. Cover out the skin of banana and slice them. Smear it with the turmeric mixture. Leave bananas in this mixture for 5-10 minutes and then drain and finally, make the chips dry.
4. Brush a little bit oil on the chips. Put them into the air fryer and cook the chips for 15 minutes.

5. Finally, mix salt and Chat Masala with this fried banana and serve immediately.

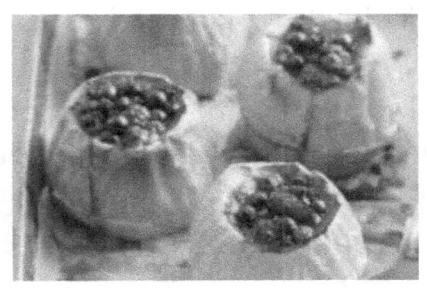

Berry Pleasure

Prep time: 10 minutes
Cook time: 18 minutes
Servings: 4

Ingredients

- 4 large apples
- ½ pound fresh strawberries
- 1 mango
- 1 cup fresh cranberries
- 2 teaspoon honey
- 1 teaspoon cinnamon
- 1 teaspoon nutmeg

- 1 teaspoon coconut oil

Directions
1. Peel and core apples, slice them.
2. Cut strawberries in half.
3. Dice the mango.
4. Combine fruits with oil.
5. Put the mixture in the air fryer and cook for 7-10 minutes at 350 F.
6. Mix honey, cinnamon and nutmeg, add to the air fryer and cook for other 4-5 minutes.

Fried Bananas with Ice Cream

Prep time: 5 minutes
Cook time: 15 minutes
Servings: 2

Ingredients
- 2 large bananas
- 1 tablespoon butter
- 1 tablespoon brown sugar
- 2 tablespoons breadcrumbs
- Vanilla ice cream for serving

Directions
1. Melt butter in the air fryer basket in one minute at 350 F

2. Mix sugar and bread crumbs in a bowl.
3. Cut bananas into 1-inch slices and add to sugar mixture. Mix well.
4. Put covered bananas into air fryer and cook for 10-15 minutes.
5. Serve warm and add ice cream.

Apple Wedges with Cinnamon

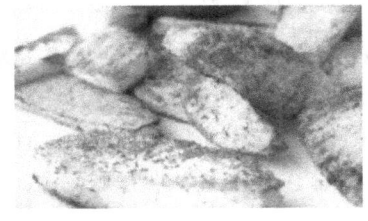

Prep time: 6 minutes
Cook time: 15 minutes
Servings: 4
Ingredients

- **4 golden apples (or as your preference)**
- **2 tablespoons sunflower oil**
- **1/2 cup dried apricots, chopped**
- **1-2 tablespoons brown sugar**
- 1/2 teaspoon ground cinnamon

Directions
1. **Peel apples and cut each one into quarters. Remove and discard cores. Cut each apple quarter in half to make 2 even wedges (each whole apple is cut into 8 even wedges).**
2. **Cover apple wedges with the oil.**
3. **Cook in the air fryer for 12-15 minutes at 350 F**
4. **Add the apricots and cook for another 3 minutes.**
5. Mix together sugar and cinnamon and top cooked apples with the sugar mixture.

Fried Bananas
Prep time: 3 minutes

Cook time: 8 minutes
Servings: 2
Ingredients
- 2 large bananas
- ½ cup plain flour
- 2 eggs, whisked
- ¾ cup breadcrumbs
- ½ cup cinnamon sugar
- 1 tablespoon olive oil
- A pinch of salt

Directions
1. Take 4 bowls and place separately: flour with salt, whisked eggs, breadcrumbs, and cinnamon sugar.
2. Peel bananas and cut them into thirds. Evenly cover bananas with the flour, then with eggs, and finally with breadcrumbs.
3. Preheat the Air Fryer to 360 F
4. Sprinkle covered bananas with olive oil and put into the air fryer. Cook for 4-5 minutes, and then make a shake to move bananas. Cook for another 4-5 minutes.

5. Remove the bananas and through then directly into the cinnamon sugar.
6. Get them cool for a minute and eat!

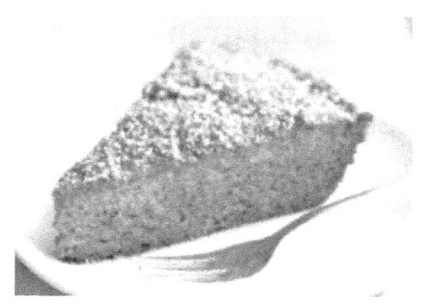

Pumpkin Cake

Prep time: 15 minutes
Cook time: 30 minutes
Servings: 4-5
Ingredients
- **1 egg**
- **6 tablespoons milk**
- **7 oz flour**
- **3 oz brown sugar**
- **5 oz pumpkin puree**
- **A pinch of salt**
- **A pinch of cinnamon (if desired)**
- Cooking spray

Directions
1. Mix pumpkin puree and brown sugar in a bowl.
2. Add one egg and whisk until smooth.
3. Mix the flour and salt. Pour milk and combine again.
4. Take the baking tin and coat with cooking spray.
5. Pour the batter into the baking tin.
6. Preheat the Air Fryer to 350 F
7. Put the baking tin to the air fryer basket and set the timer for 15 minutes.

Conclusion

Thank you for purchasing my air fryer cookbook! Hope all of the recipes from this guide were helpful and you got real pleasure and satisfaction cooking them.

Thank You

www.ingramcontent.com/pod-product-compliance
Lightning Source LLC
Chambersburg PA
CBHW052204090526
44583CB00015BA/1498